Communication Skills for Pharmacists:

Building Relationships, Improving Patient Care

Communication Skills for Pharmacists:

Building Relationships, Improving Patient Care

Bruce A. Berger, PhD, RPh
Professor of Pharmacy Care Systems
Auburn University Harrison School of Pharmacy
Auburn University, Alabama

American Pharmaceutical Association
Washington, D.C.

APhA

Editor: Nancy Tarleton Landis
Acquiring Editor: Sandra J. Cannon
Proofreader: Kathleen K. Wolter
Indexer: Suzanne Peake
Layout and Graphics: Michele A. Danoff, Graphics by Design
Cover Designer: Jim McDonald

To comment on this book via e-mail, send your message to the publisher at
aphabooks@aphanet.org.

Library of Congress Cataloging-in-Publication Data

Berger, Bruce A.
    Communication skills for pharmacists : building relationships,
improving patient care / Bruce A. Berger.
        p. ; cm.
Includes bibliographical references and index.
    ISBN 1-58212-042-0
    1. Communication in pharmacy. 2. Pharmacist and patient.
    [DNLM: 1. Pharmacy. 2. Communication. 3. Professional-Patient
Relations. QV 21 B496c 2002] I. American Pharmaceutical Association.
II. Title.

RS56 .B474 2002
615'.1—dc21
                                    2002015295

How to Order This Book
Online: www.pharmacist.com
By phone: 800-878-0729 (from the United States and Canada)
VISA®, MasterCard®, and American Express® cards accepted.

Printed in Canada

Contents

Foreword

What benefit is there from medication that is administered incorrectly? How effective is medication when patients do not understand its purpose or its side effects? Enhancing patient outcomes is a goal of pharmacists, other health care professionals, and pharmaceutical manufacturers. How is this accomplished?

We know that information on drug therapy is much needed. I believe the critical factor is the ability of all pharmacists to effectively communicate the necessary information so that patients will benefit. There is no doubt that pharmacy colleges' curricula provide the information needed to dispense the proper information with each prescription. But is the method of effective communication part of the learning experience? Is communication the delivery of correct information to every patient or caregiver? Does every person receive and understand the facts in the same way? Will they be able to interpret these facts for their own benefit?

This book is an important contribution to effective communication. The author, Dr. Bruce Berger, is a great communicator. He begins this book with a discussion of the ethical and moral responsibility of pharmacists to provide pharmaceutical care, which depends upon effective communication. In Chapter 2, Bruce discusses relationships, which can strengthen outcomes. A very important skill for effective communication is listening, which is explored in Chapter 3. Other interpersonal skills are explored in all 13 chapters. Each chapter includes discussion and thought-provoking questions. This is a must-read book. I also recommend it as a source for group discussions. It might even help you in your personal relationships with the significant others in your life.

Angèle C. D'Angelo, DSc, MS, RPh
Vice President–Editor-in-Chief
U.S. Pharmacist
June 2002

Acknowledgments

The chapters in this book are articles that were originally published in *U.S. Pharmacist*. They were adapted with the permission of Jobson Publishing, L.L.C., by author Bruce A. Berger. The American Pharmaceutical Association gratefully acknowledges the cooperation and assistance of Jobson Publishing, L.L.C., and of *U.S. Pharmacist*, Frank Bennicasa, Senior Vice President–Publisher, and Angèle C. D'Angelo, Vice President–Editor-in-Chief.

Introduction

Pharmaceutical care is the mission of pharmacy practice. It requires the development of a covenantal relationship between pharmacist and patient, in which information is exchanged, held in confidence, and used to optimize patient care through appropriate drug therapy. Developing such a relationship requires skills, hard work, and continuity of care. This book is intended to help pharmacists provide better care to patients. Its focus is the communication skills necessary to build the kind of relationships that result in improved therapeutic outcomes.

Chapter 1 sets the stage for the remainder of the book. It focuses on pharmacists' moral and ethical responsibilities in providing pharmaceutical care. In addition, this chapter discusses what it means to care, what it means to be a professional, and the roles that pharmacists, schools of pharmacy, state boards of pharmacy, and professional organizations can play in advancing the profession.

Chapter 2 discusses the need for relationships and why developing effective relationships with patients (and health care providers) is essential in the provision of pharmaceutical care. Satisfying relationships pave the way for positive treatment outcomes.

Chapter 3 introduces the skills of listening and empathic understanding. These powerful skills enable us to respond to others in a caring and respectful manner. Communicating understanding is a powerful way to help patients carry out a treatment plan.

Chapter 4 discusses principles of patient counseling and how counseling differs from simply providing information. The chapter includes a checklist, with a detailed explanation, that pharmacists can use in counseling patients about their medications.

Even when pharmacists use their best interpersonal skills, patients or health care providers may still become angry and direct that anger at the pharmacist. **Chapter 5** discusses how to deal with anger effectively. To maintain therapeutic relationships, we need to understand this strong and powerful emotion and respond to it appropriately.

Chapter 6 presents the basic tenets of assertiveness and skills involved in becoming assertive. It distinguishes assertive, nonassertive, and aggressive behaviors and explores rights and responsibilities in assertive communication.

Conflict in relationships is inevitable. As long as people hold differing values, conflicts will occur. The way we manage conflicts can promote understanding—or undermine the relationship. **Chapter 7** discusses effective and ineffective ways of managing conflict.

Pharmaceutical care requires a dramatic change in pharmacists' practice. Taking medications and adjusting one's lifestyle to manage a chronic illness also requires change. **Chapter 8** explores change and how to help patients manage the changes necessary to effectively control an illness. Applications of the transtheoretical model of change and motivational interviewing are discussed.

Pharmaceutical care cannot be provided effectively without productive relationships with physicians. **Chapter 9** discusses how to call a physician and how to have a face-to-face conversation when drug therapy problems arise.

Chapter 10 explores supportive communication. Different emotions, such as anger, sadness, and anxiety, have different origins. A response that soothes an angry patient may not be appropriate for a patient who is depressed after learning about a chronic condition. Different types of responses are needed if communication is to be caring and effective.

Chapter 11 summarizes types of responses and when each is appropriate and effective. For example, pharmacists need to discern when it is appropriate to give advice and when it is not.

Chapter 12 examines persuasive communication. It describes conditions in which persuasive communication can be effective and times when it is not only ineffective but can actually cause more resistance.

Chapter 13 provides examples of immediate and nonimmediate verbal and nonverbal communication. Both what we say and how we say it can affect whether we are perceived as caring, aloof, involved, or indifferent.

Chapter 1
CARING, COVENANTS, CODES, AND COMMITMENT

We are facing massive change in health care in general and pharmacy in particular. The pharmacy profession is changing much more rapidly now than it was 5 years ago, yet many pharmacists are still fighting change rather than embracing it. Many in the profession are looking for someone to blame rather than deciding how to move forward.

> Pharmaceutical care requires the development of a covenantal relationship with our patients. It requires that we care and provide care.

Pharmacy has responded to changes in the health care system in part by making pharmaceutical care its mission. Pharmaceutical care requires completely rethinking the way pharmacists have traditionally practiced. Some pharmacists confuse it with patient counseling or disease management, but pharmaceutical care is far more complex and offers many more challenges.

Pharmaceutical care requires that pharmacists take responsibility for preventing and solving drug-related problems and optimizing drug therapy. This means that real and potential problems must be identified and solved by talking to and working with patients and other health care providers. This does not end when the patient leaves the pharmacy. Assessing, monitoring, documenting care and progress, and follow-up care are integral parts of providing pharmaceutical care. And assessing means not just physical assessment of the patient but assessment of the patient's understanding of the illness and the treatment plan. Pharmaceutical care also means involving the patient throughout the process.

In addition, pharmaceutical care requires marketing and management support. No doubt, there is a market need for pharmaceutical care, but there is not yet a clear market demand. Patients don't know they need it, physicians aren't sure what it is or if they should like it, and payers don't understand it or aren't convinced that it will really reduce health care costs. As I've traveled throughout the United States, Canada, and Australia discussing pharmaceutical care with pharmacists, I've heard a common theme. Most pharmacists *are* convinced that we must make the transition to pharmaceutical care for the sake of our patients and our profession. Most also agree that there is a market need but not a market demand. But few see it as their job to create this demand—to "sell" pharmaceutical care and the mission of pharmacy. We are waiting for someone else to sell our mission. But only pharmacists really care about pharmacy, so it is up to every pharmacist to market pharmaceutical care. And we need to start now.

This chapter provides observations about the profession of pharmacy, the problems it faces, and some solutions for a productive and exciting future. I don't want to sound pessimistic, but I don't believe many in the profession will survive without embracing the changes we face. Dispensing drugs alone won't cut it. The health care system has sent a clear message to pharmacy that simply dispensing drugs has very little value. In fact, drugs dispensed without proper education and involvement substantially raise health care costs. We don't need more studies to prove this last point. The only real argument is whether we are talking about $75 billion, $100 billion, or $150 billion in health care costs resulting from drug-related morbidity and mortality.

The health care system has also told us quite clearly that it won't pay for anything that doesn't lower costs or improve outcomes. Yet many pharmacists continue to cling to dispensing, even as fees and reimbursement for drug costs shrink. Some argue that they have no time to do anything but dispense drugs and that, furthermore, they don't get paid to do anything else. But they cannot afford to *not* make the time, and why would people pay for services they are not yet getting? I am certainly not saying that pharmacists should give up control of dispensing. I am simply saying that we must be more involved in the care of the patient.

Rethinking Our Standard of Care

Some time ago I went to a pharmacy with a new prescription. The pharmacist was alone and the pharmacy was not busy. The pharmacist filled my prescription, attached an information leaflet to the stapled bag, and collected my copayment. Then he held out a clipboard with a pad of two-column, lined paper on it, pointed to the right-hand column of the pad, and said, "Sign here," pointing to the line below several previous signatures. I asked to see the clipboard, and as I looked through the pages I noticed that all the previous signatures were in the right-hand column. In small print at the top of that column was the statement "I do not want counseling" and, at the top of the left-hand column, "I want counseling." I was never asked whether I wanted counseling or if I had any questions before I was instructed to "Sign here." I never received any verbal (spoken) counseling. I looked at the pharmacist and said, "What you are doing is illegal. But worse than that, it is immoral and unethical. You have asked me to sign a waiver of my right to informed consent without informing me of what I am giving up, all so that you don't have to verbally offer to counsel me about my medicine. I am going to report you to the state board."

The pharmacist was aghast as he looked at me and said, "Why? What are you talking about? It's not my fault."

"Whose fault is it?" I asked.

He said, "My district manager wants us to do this."

I looked at him and said, "This is truly sad. Your obligation is to me, not to your district manager. You are here to serve the public—to protect me. You are licensed by privilege, not by right. Whenever we allow others to dictate our standards, we, in a very real sense, lose our profession."

As I walked away, he said, "I can't believe this."

I cannot say for certain that I would be different if I were practicing pharmacy. I wish I could say that this was an isolated incident in pharmacy. It was not. I felt obligated to report this pharmacist because of my own professional duty. It *is* my obligation to police my own profession. Pharmacists have an obligation to report this kind of behavior. It not only puts the public at risk, it hurts all of us professionally.

In times of chaotic change, like that occurring in pharmacy, people and organizations may behave in ways and make decisions that are not consistent with how they would behave under less stressful conditions—sometimes at the expense of the clients they are supposed to serve and protect. When faced with the problems created by chaotic change, people respond in one of three ways: they "go numb," blame someone else, or solve the problem.

The pharmacist I encountered was ready to blame someone else. He clearly did not understand what it meant to be a professional, to care about me as the patient more than about the employer who was asking him to put people at risk. It is easy to blame the employer, but the real problem lies with the pharmacist. Granted, it would take great courage to stand up as a professional and say, "In good conscience, I cannot ask patients to sign this. I won't do it." But that is exactly what we need to do: to say that *we* control our profession's standards, not anyone else. Because pharmacists are in short supply, we have the leverage to say, "Keep your signing bonuses and car leases. I want 8 to 16 hours of uninterrupted time each week to schedule patient care."

What Do We Know about Our Patients?

What has happened to the pharmacy profession? How did we get here? We have lost sight of what is truly important: the patient. We are licensed by privilege to make sure that the drugs patients receive are appropriate for each individual patient. That means we need to know something about our patients. What does the patient know and understand about the illness and its treatment? Does the patient believe the diagnosis? What's a typical day like for the patient? To what extent do patients intend to take responsibility for their illnesses? Do they understand what they have been told and the choices available to them?

When we practice pharmacy, are we able to answer these questions? If the answer is no, then why *don't* we know these things? We say that pharmaceutical care is our mission, but is it our standard? Can people expect to receive pharmaceutical care in every pharmacy where they present a prescription or when they need information about treating an illness? What can the profession promise and deliver in every pharmacy in the United States? Are we, collectively, delivering more than just the drug the physician ordered? The answer is no. Why, then, do we expect to get paid for more when our national standard is to only dispense the drug? Clearly, some pharmacists are delivering more, but they are not in the majority.

Are we behaving morally and ethically as a profession? When patients do not receive important information about their medication, and when we do not assess their understanding of the illness and treatment, we are putting them at risk. When we ask patients to sign a waiver of their right to counseling, to circumvent the intent of OBRA '90,[a] we are depriving them of their right to informed consent—their right to make informed decisions about the medications they are about to take (or not take). Again, we are putting them at risk. We say we don't have time and we aren't paid for this (and because many other pharmacies do the same, it must be all right), but none of these reasons make it right.

Caring

Pharmaceutical care requires the development of a covenantal relationship with our patients. It requires that we care and provide care. The first principle of the American Pharmaceutical Association (APhA) Code of Ethics states, "A pharmacist respects the covenantal relationship between the patient and pharmacist." What does this mean? Why is it important? What is caring? What are covenantal relationships? What do these concepts have to do with our code of ethics and the need for our profession to commit itself to these concepts?

Pharmaceutical care is "the responsible provision of drug therapy for the purpose of achieving definite outcomes that improve a patient's quality of life."[1] According to Hepler and Strand,[1] "There are four criteria to be considered before pharmacists should be granted authority or pharmacists should accept responsibility for

---

[a]*The Omnibus Budget Reconciliation Act of 1990. This law contains the Medicaid Prescription Drug Reform Act, which mandates drug-use review and patient counseling—or the offer to counsel—for all outpatient prescriptions covered by Medicaid. Most states now have such counseling requirements for all patients.*

providing pharmaceutical care: (i) the provider must possess knowledge and skill in pharmaceutics and clinical pharmacology; (ii) the provider must be able to mobilize the drug distribution system by which drug use decisions are implemented; (iii) *the provider must be able to develop the relationships with the patient and other health care professionals needed to provide pharmaceutical care*; and (iv) as a practical matter, the provider must be available in society in sufficient numbers."

Pharmaceutical care requires a much more intimate and intensive relationship between the pharmacist and patient. Information must be provided and understood by both the patient and the pharmacist. Problems the patient has now or has had with medications must be explored in a manner that is nonjudgmental and nonthreatening. Appropriate medication regimens must be tailored to the needs of the individual patient, not the needs of the provider. Concerns that patients have about their illness or treatment must be addressed in a way that legitimizes, not minimizes, the concerns. That is, pharmaceutical care requires caring. But what does caring mean?

At the most basic level, caring means attending to the needs of others—making the concerns of others paramount:[2]

> When we have genuinely received another, we often feel our motive energy flowing toward the needs and projects of the other. We want to help—to relieve pain, to achieve a goal that is not our own, to actualize a dream. This is a feeling that all carers experience when they are in an authentic caring mode. The self is still there with all its own ideals, loves, and projects, but its energy is temporarily put into the service of the other's needs.

Carl Rogers[3] would call this unconditional positive regard. This is the willingness to be loving and accepting of the patient. When pharmacists make themselves available to patients, they relieve some of their patients' sense of fear and loneliness. This is the work of empathic understanding. The questions the pharmacist must ask are, "Can I permit myself to enter into the private world of my patients, explore their feelings without judging them, and, in some significant and honest way, respond in a manner that lets them know that I have listened and I want to provide whatever assistance or comfort that I can? Can I see this person as having a unique reaction to his or her illness? Can I learn enough about this person so that the insight or assistance I give is likely to be useful?"

Reich[4] stated that "care means worry or concern.... The significance of this meaning of care is that if nothing matters, if nothing is worth worrying about, ethics is not possible. Any attempt to develop a systematic inquiry into the moral life would be bogged down, for the moral life itself would be mired in apathy." What Reich is saying is that only when I care about something or someone do I transcend my own self-oriented desires and develop morality. In fact, this is one of the first lessons we try to teach children: to care about others, to see and be concerned about the impact of what they do and how the choices they make affect others.

Ethics and morality depend on caring about the welfare of others. In fact, ethical decision-making involves identifying which issues (of many) are the most salient or important for my attention and concern. What merits my moral caring or concern? For example, pharmacists may say they do not have time (or do not get paid) to render pharmaceutical care. If a patient came to your pharmacy and you knew that the drug prescribed would kill the patient, given the patient's prior medical history, would you intervene despite how busy you were and whether you got paid? I hope so. What if the medication would "only" blind the patient? Would you still intervene despite time and money? Again, I hope so. What if the medication would cause explosive diarrhea that would hospitalize the patient within 3 days? Less certain about intervening? I hope not. The point is that we must decide what caring behavior is. What are the most salient issues here? Time? Money? The degree of risk the patient will assume? Why do we think we have the right to decide the extent to which the patient will be at risk or how much harm is sufficient to intervene? These are issues of care and concern for the value of human life. Becoming a professional, by definition, means that what we do is not solely motivated by financial gain. In fact, the primary motivation is service to the public. You might say that this is altruistic. I would argue that the foundation for professional behavior *is* altruism.

Professionalism

What are the characteristics of a professional? How would we recognize one if we saw one? Consider the following characteristics:

Expertise. This results from prolonged and intensive specialized training. It is unique expertise that allows the professional the power to make decisions about the client. The client grants this authority

> **R**
>
> **Characteristics of a Professional**
>
> - Expertise
> - Autonomy
> - Identification with the profession
> - Commitment to a calling
> - Ethics
> - Collegial maintenance of standards

to the professional because of the unique expertise. The client also assumes that the professional will use this power to serve the client, not the needs of the professional.

Autonomy. This involves self-control over decisions and work activities, motivated by doing what is right for the client. It also involves a commitment to providing clients sufficient information so that they can make better decisions about their own well-being. But it does not stop with simply providing information. There is an advocacy role here, one of patient empowerment. Patient advocacy involves more than giving patients information in order to satisfy their right to informed consent or autonomy. Advocacy is more than giving patients what they want. Giving a patient information without assessing the patient's understanding of that information is a form of paternalism, in which the health care provider decides what is enough. Moreover, health care providers should not leave patients alone in decisions about managing their health, believing that giving patients information is all that the job requires. We cannot leave it to the patient to sort through a maze of information and decide what is best. This simply won't work, and it is not true advocacy and does not promote empowerment.

So what is true advocacy? Existential advocacy, according to Gadow,[5] involves "participation with the patient in determining the unique meaning which the experience of health, illness, suffering, or dying is to have for that individual." Gadow elaborates:

> The ideal which existential advocacy expresses is this: that individuals be *assisted...to authentically* exercise their freedom of self-determination. By authentic is meant a way of reaching decisions which are truly one's own— decisions that express all that one believes important about oneself and the world, the entire complexity of one's values.

To do this, patients must not only be informed about their illnesses and treatment options, but they must also be given ample opportunity to express their understanding, beliefs, and values about the illness and treatment options. They must be given the time and encouragement to ask questions, raise concerns, and express feelings about what is happening to them. The health care provider does not leave patients in isolation to decide on their own. The health care provider can help by expressing what he or she thinks is advisable, but ultimately all decisions must be up to the patient. This kind of advocacy values the patient's right to self-determination above all other human rights; it is essential to patient empowerment.

Identification with the profession. Professionals take pride in their profession. They want the profession to thrive, not merely survive. They hold the profession to high standards and attempt to raise the standards of the profession.

Commitment to a calling. Professionals are committed to their careers and to lifelong learning. They are committed to staying current because they know this is necessary in order to serve patients and maintain the expertise that allowed patients to entrust them with power in the first place.

Ethics. Professions have internal codes of ethics. Why? Because the public is not in a position to determine whether professional standards are being met. Codes are a written and public commitment to serve and protect the public as consistent with the expertise of the professional. But no profession should develop a code of ethics without input from the public the profession serves. Failure to seek such input would indicate that the profession presumes to know what is best for the public—to know this better than the public itself. This is simply another form of paternalism. Why would a professional with expertise in pharmacotherapy presume to know what is best for a patient's life (e.g., for the patient's family life and daily routines)? The expertise does not qualify the professional to know that.

Collegial maintenance of standards. This means that professionals are committed to policing themselves. Again, because the general public often does not know if standards are being met, professionals must police themselves in order to make good on their promise to serve and protect the public. For example, many patients do not know or understand what OBRA '90 requires of the pharmacy or pharmacist. Some pharmacists are asking patients to waive their right to counseling but not informing them about what they are waiving. This has the potential to harm patients. It certainly does not serve them. Pharmacists who know this is going on are obligated to report it to protect patients.

Professionalism implies the use of expertise to serve the public need:[6]

Professionals develop a public and moral responsibility to others by internalizing a clear sense of purpose, a strong commitment to serve the public, and a deep understanding of the ethic of the profession. This professional responsibility is reflected in the way professionals behave toward their clients and toward each other.

This is why professional decisions must not be tempered by time or money. That is, pharmacists cannot use "I don't have time" or "I don't get paid" as an excuse for neglecting basic duties to the patient. I am fully in favor of professionals being paid for their expertise. Their expertise is the capital they have to sell. I am simply saying that to truly be a professional mandates that one *not require* payment to provide needed services. This is altruism and is part of the definition of a professional. This is a risk we are willing to take to become a professional.

Covenants

Recall that pharmaceutical care requires the development of a covenantal relationship with our patients. What does this mean? A covenant is a promise. It is a gift. It is something owed. What do we owe patients? We owe them our expertise. We owe them sufficient time and energy to allow them to understand their illness and its treatment and to ask questions about those things and choices they don't understand or are unclear about. We owe them current information and the highest quality standards we can provide. We owe it to them to ask ourselves, "How would God (or whoever your purveyor of truth is) practice pharmacy?" and "Would God (or your purveyor of truth) practice pharmacy the way I am practicing it?" If the answer to either question indicates that we are far from where we need to be, let us not beat ourselves up. Let us begin the work of figuring out how to get where we know we should be, no matter how difficult the task, no matter how many roadblocks are thrown in front of us, because it is simply the right thing to do. More on this later.

In her courageous talk at the American Society of Health-System Pharmacists leadership conference in 1999, Kathleen Marie Dixon[7] called upon pharmacists to take up the torch of virtue theory and ethics. She reminded us that the ethicist Philippa Foot said, "For sometimes one man succeeds where another fails not because there is some specific difference in their previous conduct but because his heart lies in a different place; and the disposition of the heart is part of virtue." Dixon went on to say that virtue theory helps us to re-engage our hearts in both our work and our selves. She referred to

a spark of passion, perhaps not for the discipline as it is practiced today, but for what it *can be*. That perception of excellence, that insight into virtue, grounds this paradigm. That spark can pass quickly between human beings, creating interest in and desire for personal development, revealing new patterns of thought and experience. This in turn becomes the engine that drives professional change.

Dixon is talking about doing what you already know is right.

Codes

In 1994 the profession of pharmacy, spearheaded by APhA and encouraged by the Joint Commission of Pharmacy Practitioners, put forth a new and dramatically different Code of Ethics. The Code is based on the concept of pharmaceutical care as developed by Hepler and Strand.[1] It requires a level of professional practice that carries with it far more responsibilities, yet far more autonomy. Votterro[8] commented that "Pharmacists who respond to this additional level of professional practice and autonomy and embrace the unique *caring* expectations of this new practice mode will be further challenged to demonstrate group and personal behavior that may be far beyond the present expectations of society." The preamble and eight principles of the Code of Ethics for Pharmacists appear in the sidebar on page 10, and the full text of the Code[9] is available at www.aphanet.org/pharmcare/ethics.html.

Look at the first principle: "A pharmacist respects the covenantal relationship between the patient and pharmacist." There is that covenant thing again. Are we

Code of Ethics for Pharmacists

Preamble

Pharmacists are health professionals who assist individuals in making the best use of medications. This Code, prepared and supported by pharmacists, is intended to state publicly the principles that form the fundamental basis of the roles and responsibilities of pharmacists. These principles, based on moral obligations and virtues, are established to guide pharmacists in relationships with patients, health professionals, and society.

I. A pharmacist respects the covenantal relationship between the patient and pharmacist.
II. A pharmacist promotes the good of every patient in a caring, compassionate, and confidential manner.
III. A pharmacist respects the autonomy and dignity of each patient.
IV. A pharmacist acts with honesty and integrity in professional relationships.
V. A pharmacist maintains professional competence.
VI. A pharmacist respects the values and abilities of colleagues and other health professionals.
VII. A pharmacist serves individual, community, and societal needs.
VIII. A pharmacist seeks justice in the distribution of health resources.

Adopted by the membership of the American Pharmaceutical Association October 27, 1994.

serious about this? This is a profoundly important statement. What it requires of the pharmacist is serious business. It requires a commitment on the part of the pharmacist to virtues and existential advocacy. Are we ready? Are we to have a Code in name only—something that is nice but that we really don't intend to do—or is it time to seriously challenge ourselves and ask, How do we get there? How do we make our Code live? If we are not ready, what steps are needed to get us there?

Standards

To move forward, we must look at standards. What is pharmacy's standard? What can we promise patients when they walk into a pharmacy to get a prescription filled? Do pharmacists provide verbal counseling for each patient with a new prescription? Do pharmacists provide all patients with written medication information? In both cases, the answer is no. What we generally *do* provide for each patient is the medication ordered by the physician. We are very good at dispensing exactly what is written on the prescription. Unfortunately, what the physician orders is not always appropriate for the patient.

There *are* many pharmacists who counsel each patient and not only question the appropriateness of the drug therapy prescribed but also act on the behalf of patients to change the drug therapy when necessary. However, for this to be a standard, it must be done each time, by all pharmacists. That is what a standard of practice is. Why are we surprised that we get paid (and often not well) only for dispensing drugs, when that is our standard? Pharmacists who have raised their standard are getting paid for more than just dispensing.

So, how do we develop standards? One way is to look at what we know. What does research tell us about what must happen to produce positive drug therapy outcomes? We know that in order to achieve optimal outcomes from their drug therapy, patients must

Understand the diagnosis. Do patients understand the diagnosis and treatment? Do they know what they need to do? Do they believe they can do it?

Be interested in their health. Do patients care whether or not they get healthier, and do they want to prevent illness?

Correctly assess the potential impact of the diagnosis. Do patients understand what will happen if they do or do not treat the illness appropriately?

Believe in the efficacy of the prescribed treatment. Do patients believe that the medication will have the intended effect? Do they understand what the medication actually does and how they will know whether it is working?

Find ways of using the medication that are not more trouble than the disease. Some illnesses "feel" better than the treatment. For example, patients with high blood pressure often initially feel worse when they are put on medication. Do they understand that this may happen? Do they know that this is usually transient? Do they know what to do if this condition does not change after a specified period of time? Do patients know how long it should take for the medicine to have its intended effect, what the effect is, and how to measure it, if necessary (e.g., by measuring blood pressure or peak flow)?

Be assessed regarding their readiness. Substantial literature supports variation among patients in readiness to manage their illnesses and the self-management behaviors necessary to manage the illness. Different strategies are necessary for different stages of readiness. Are patients being properly assessed so that appropriate interventions are used?

Patients who meet these criteria are likely to adhere to (comply with) their medication regimens. Therefore, if pharmacists are to have a substantive impact on health outcomes in patients, our standards of practice must include ways of addressing these issues. The way we communicate information to patients is part of our standards. For example, how do we tell patients what "1 bid" means? Do we tell them that this means approximately 12 hours apart and then tailor the dosing times to their daily routine, or do we tell them to take the medicine twice a day and hope they figure out what we mean? What does "1 pc and hs" mean? What does it mean for a patient with diabetes who eats six small meals a day? Do we really want him taking the medicine seven times a day? *How* we communicate information should be part of our standards, because it affects treatment outcomes.

Making the Transition: Some Assumptions

Before going any further, it is important to state some underlying assumptions:

- Pharmaceutical care is the mission of pharmacy practice. It involves optimizing health outcomes through the appropriate use of pharmacotherapy.
- There is a market need for pharmaceutical care. Pharmacists must create the demand.
- Most pharmacists want to provide pharmaceutical care. Many have a hard time imagining how to do so in an environment that has focused on dispensing drugs.
- Providing pharmaceutical care will lower health care costs in total (or at the very least, raise quality without increasing the total costs of care).
- Great courage is needed by all pharmacists in all work settings to demand that our professional standards *not* be compromised. What is courage? It is the will to look for right answers. According to Dixon,[7] "What brings the right answer is an exercise of justice and realism and really looking. The difficulty is to keep the attention fixed upon the real situation and to prevent focusing on our own needs or defenses."
- Pharmacists need not fear that they will lose their jobs for upholding the law or raising standards.
- We must stop blaming others for our problems. When people are placed in extraordinary or difficult situations in which they must choose that which is good, right, or moral versus that which is expedient, great courage is needed. Otherwise they must become numb or blame someone or something else in order to escape the pain of giving up what they know is right. Pharmacists, for far too long now, have been placed in those very difficult situations in which they must choose, and too often they have chosen what is expedient. To be courageous is very frightening and often painfully lonely. However, doing what we know at our core is just not right hurts our very souls. That is a much higher price to pay, and it is time for it to stop.
- We must stop believing that anyone other than pharmacists is interested in our survival as a profession.

■ The transition will require a concerted effort from many different groups, including pharmacists, schools of pharmacy and their faculty members, pharmacy students, state boards of pharmacy, providers of continuing professional education, and our state and national professional associations.

What Pharmacists Can Do

Let's start with what pharmacists need to do. First, we must realize that whenever members of a profession allow others to dictate their practice standards, they, in a very real sense, cease to be a profession. Pharmacists must be willing to do the courageous work of standing up and saying that something is terribly wrong when their professional ethics and morals are compromised. What would this mean? It would mean actively counseling patients regardless of how busy you are. It would mean that patients would, at minimum, be assessed to ensure that the medication prescribed is right for them and to make sure they understand their illness and its treatment, and that they would have their questions or concerns addressed (or an appointment would be made to do so).

Impossible, you say. Patients would get backed up. Patients would find another pharmacy to go to because they wouldn't want to wait. Many would call corporate offices complaining about the long waits. You could get fired. Or, for the first time, patients would see how valuable the pharmacist is and would be willing to wait for and pay for this value (we know that patients consistently say they want and value this from the pharmacist).

Some patients would leave and go where it's cheap and fast. Some would call corporate offices and complain. What are we afraid of? Do we really believe that someone is going to fire a pharmacist for raising or upholding standards? If a pharmacist did get fired for this, I think the pharmacist would have a case to successfully sue the organization.

Best of all, *we*, not some external body, would be setting our standards. The danger is, of course, that few would be brave enough to do this. But what a day this would be! Jesse Vivian, a pharmacist and attorney, has said he would welcome the opportunity to defend any pharmacist who is fired for upholding or raising standards.

Start small. I challenge you to identify one patient in your pharmacy each month for whom you will provide a high level of care. It could be a patient with asthma or diabetes that is not well controlled. It may require coming in 20 minutes early for your shift or staying 20 minutes late (or whatever it takes). Document the care you provide and, with the patient's permission, provide the documentation to the patient's primary care physician, the patient, the patient's employer, and the patient's third-party payer, and send the payer an invoice for your services. The patient's physician needs to know there is a pharmacy in town where this level of care is provided. This could be a great source of referrals.

Promote this service when you are ready. The message to general practitioners (GPs) and family practitioners (FPs) should be, "If we work together to keep Mrs. X's diabetes [for example] under control, you get to keep the patient." In other words, the GP or FP doesn't lose the patient to a specialist, such as an endocrinologist or pulmonologist. Moreover, many pharmacists report that they have now engaged physicians in writing prescriptions for care. For example, the physician writes an order for diabetes education and monitoring. This order is attached to the documentation and to the invoice sent to the third-party payer as justification for the service.

The patient should get a copy of the documentation so he or she is aware of what you have done. The employer should get a copy because, ultimately, employers pay for health care in the United States. Furthermore, this speaks volumes about the level of care a local pharmacist can provide, and employers can use this information in deciding whether to use local pharmacies or a mail order service.

Think about this. There are approximately 150,000 practicing pharmacists in the United States. If, once each month, only one-third of those pharmacists submitted documentation for compensation for services rendered to a single patient with a chronic illness, the profession collectively would provide third parties with over 50,000 pieces of evidence that this is not an isolated way of practicing. Our standard would be raised, and the profession would be in a much better position to negotiate compensation for patient care services. Initially, would everyone get paid? Probably not. Would someone? Some already are. To see who some of them are, go to the Auburn University Pharmacy Care Systems Web site (http://pharmacy.auburn.edu/pcs). Click on "Innovative Pharmacy Practitioners," then choose a category from the Innovator Menu. Or, go to the APhA Web site (www.aphanet.org). Click on "Pharmaceutical Care" in the far left column, then click on the "Pharmaceutical Care Networking Directory" and follow the instructions.

Every successful innovative practitioner started by changing his or her practice with a single patient. And successful innovators will all tell you the same thing: It is not the money that now keeps them going. It is their own sense that what they are doing is valuable and meaningful to the patients they are serving. They go home knowing they have helped someone.

What should you do if you *are* paid? Don't keep it to yourself. Tell us at Auburn or at APhA, and we will put you on our Web site. Write up your success story for your local or state pharmacy journal or newsletter, and share what you have learned so that others can follow your example.

> **When pharmacists make themselves available to patients, they relieve some of their patients' sense of fear and loneliness.**

If you are an employee pharmacist in a corporate pharmacy, ask your district manager for permission to identify a patient or a handful of patients with whom you can work more intensively as a pilot project. You may have to donate some of your time at first. But let the corporation know that if there is compensation by the patient or a third party, you want to share the rewards, through either higher compensation or more help (e.g., people, technology), so that you can expand what you are doing.

Develop a patient promise. Years ago, Folgers sold millions of dollars worth of coffee by telling consumers that Folgers was "mountain grown." Of course, this was the truth, but it was also true for every other quality coffee on the market. Folgers simply took a fact about coffee and paired it with the attribute of quality to get consumers to believe that mountain-grown Folgers was best. It worked.

What does this have to do with pharmacy? There are so many things you do on a daily basis for your patients that you take for granted. Your patients often do not appreciate these things because they simply don't know about them. For example, do you make sure the drug dispensed is not outdated? That it is the right quantity and strength? That it will not cause problems with any other medications or illnesses the patient may have? Do you provide a set of information (verbally or otherwise) to the patient with each new prescription dispensed that contains the name of the drug, strength, directions for use, precautions, major side effects, and so on?

To develop a patient promise, make a list on your pharmacy's letterhead of everything you do or provide for patients each time they get a prescription filled in your pharmacy. Include all of the things I have already listed and anything else you do each time. Do not promise things you don't do each time. Also list additional services that are available upon request. Whenever a patient gets a new prescription filled, hand the patient your sheet and say, "I don't know what other pharmacies in town do, but this is what I will do for you each time you get a new prescription filled here. [Remember 'mountain grown.'] If you have any questions, please let me know."

Create a demand for needed services. How do you do this? The next time a patient walks in with a new prescription for high blood pressure, for example, look at the patient and say,

Mr. Smith, you have high blood pressure. I want to make sure that this medicine lowers your blood pressure to the point where you are not at risk for a stroke or a heart attack. The only way we can know that your medicine is really working is to monitor your blood pressure. You simply can't feel when your blood pressure is up or down. You will see your doctor only every 3 to 6 months, and I don't want to wait that long to be sure that your medicine is working properly for you. I can offer you blood pressure monitoring equipment and teach you how to use it; I sell several types. Or, I have a blood pressure monitoring service for which I charge $X per month. You would come in as often as you would like, but at least once a week, and I would keep track of your blood pressure and send your doctor your readings every 2 weeks so we can work together to keep you as healthy as possible. Which do you prefer?

What's the worst the patient can say? "I don't want either." At least you would have offered a needed service and expressed your caring and concern. This would take all of 45 seconds. The same could be done with asthma and peak flow meters or diabetes monitoring if allowed in your state. Develop an herbal remedy consultation service. If people are willing to spend hundreds of dollars in a health food store, are they willing to pay to have you assess their nutritional and nutraceuticals needs in a systematic, scientific way? And who better to do this than a pharmacist? What do you have to lose?

Re-evaluate your practice. This means everything: the physical environment, the workflow, technology, products sold, who does what, and so on. Are you performing tasks a technician can do? Do you sell products or services that have nothing to do with health care and may, in fact, be contrary to good health (e.g., tobacco products, beer, wine)? What messages are you sending to consumers about the business you are in? What do your patients want and need? When is the last time you asked them? What do physicians in your area need and want? Have you done any physician detailing to promote new services in collaboration with a physician? Have you discussed services you would like to provide with physicians in your area? Have you asked them what services they need? Have you tried speaking at a local medical association meeting? Have you tried speaking at a local PTA meeting about such things as seasonal services?

Think outside the box. Don't limit your practice or what you do to a physical site. This includes counseling and other services. If the service is needed, take the mountain to Muhammad: Make house calls. Make telephone calls. Counseling can be done by phone. Learn to think creatively about what patients want and how to provide it. Have you gotten involved in e-business? Do you have a Web presence? What do you use it for? Do your patients know about it? How can it help them? Are you brick-and-click or brick or click only? Do you know what this means? If not, you need more help from experts.

Upgrade or refresh your skills. Attend certificate programs offered by your state and national pharmacy associations, schools of pharmacy, or other organizations. Become an expert in a disease such as diabetes or asthma. Offer services to support disease management and charge for them. Become a smoking-cessation expert. Go out and seek expertise in whatever excites your passion and promotes a higher standard of care. When you go for additional training in disease management, for example, stay in touch with the others who have been trained so that you can share successes and problems. Before leaving the training session, be sure someone is developing a workgroup or listserv through e-mail. That way, all of you can stay in touch and ask each other how problems with implementation, patient acceptance, payment, and so on are being resolved. Not having the support of others has been a critical barrier to implementing new service offerings.

Develop mentoring sites. Develop sites throughout your state where innovative practice is occurring, and use those sites as mentoring or apprenticeship sites. If your site is one of those, charge other pharmacists for this apprenticeship training. It is valuable, and we must stop giving away our value.

What Schools of Pharmacy Can Do

It is vital to understand that pharmaceutical care requires the development of problem-solving skills and abilities on the part of practitioners. A pharmacist must be able to anticipate, prevent, and solve drug-related problems; prioritize which problems need to be attended to first (in cooperation with the patient); develop action plans that include alternatives (including nondrug therapies); and justify these alternatives to patients, physicians, and third parties. This requires skills different from those needed to dispense prescriptions. Students must be exposed to patient care early on and throughout their pharmacy school experience.

In addition, different teaching methods are needed. The accreditation standards of the American Council on Pharmaceutical Education have clearly spelled out competency areas and the need for new teaching methods and assessment techniques, but faculty members, like anyone else faced with change, have been somewhat reluctant to embrace many of these changes.

Arguments have been made, in the name of academic freedom, for the right to teach "what I want and how I want." Of course, this is not at all what academic freedom is about. Courses and course objectives are determined by the faculty as a whole, not by an individual course instructor. A faculty member has the academic freedom to choose teaching means or methods that support the course objectives. Academic freedom does not allow a faculty member to lecture because he or she is more comfortable with lecturing, if this teaching method does not support course objectives. For example, a lecture is not sufficient for meeting the following objective: "The student shall be able to demonstrate caring and understanding." This objective requires active, not passive, participation on the part of the student, through role-playing, group work, and so on. For students to demonstrate the ability to identify and prioritize drug-related problems and their solutions, more than a lecture is required. Thus, the provision of pharmaceutical care requires faculty members to incorporate different teaching methods, such as problem-based learning and small group participation. To do anything less than this is not responsible.

Another area that needs to be revisited in schools of pharmacy is admissions criteria. We need to measure more than just prepharmacy grade point average (GPA). We need to look at indexes or validated scales that measure communication abilities and traits such as extroversion and introversion. Interviews should be developed that assess caring skills (or desire), what research the applicant has done to learn about changes in the profession, and the applicant's problem-solving abilities. We need to attract people to the profession who can do more than just pass a class. We need people who care about people and what happens to them. As the profession changes and what pharmacists can do becomes more visible to the public, pharmacy school admissions screening will become easier.

Several years ago, a colleague and I did a study of communication apprehension and shyness in pharmacy students compared with nursing students. We found that one-fifth to one-fourth of pharmacy students were severely apprehensive about communicating and one-third were shy. These numbers are higher than population averages. Only one-seventh of nursing students were severely apprehensive about communicating, and just over one-tenth were shy. Why does nursing attract people who are less apprehensive and less shy than pharmacy students and the population in general? Probably because it is clearer that a person going into nursing will have to be directly involved in patient care, touching the patient, talking to the patient one-on-one, and so on. In community pharmacy, sufficient barriers still distance the pharmacist from the patient; this may be attractive to someone who wants to be in a health profession but is uncomfortable about communicating. As pharmacists' patient care activities become more visible, the profession will attract people who are less communication apprehensive and less shy.

Schools need to become far more serious about developing professional attitudes and behaviors on the part of our students. This is not magic. It takes work. Becoming a professional is a socialization process. We expect our students to act like professionals, to become professionals, simply because we have admitted them. Often, there is no formal process in place to make sure this actually occurs. We need to identify the attitudes and behaviors we expect and why these attitudes and behaviors are necessary and important, and then put the appropriate structure in place to make sure this occurs. I find it repugnant that we graduate individuals with great GPAs who couldn't care less what happens to a patient. We have put a number of things in place to address this concern: an honor code, a professional development committee, an extensive orientation for new students, and pharmacy practice experiences. We have a long way to go, but we are making progress.

Pharmaceutical care requires *care*. We need to teach our students about

> The transition [to pharmaceutical care] will require a concerted effort from many different groups, including pharmacists, schools of pharmacy and their faculty members, pharmacy students, state boards of pharmacy, providers of continuing professional education, and our state and national professional associations.

patient caring and the skills that go with that. We need to change how they think about patients. If we wait until their last year in school to expose them to patients, it is too little too late. The day our students are admitted they are assigned a patient. They are also assigned to two faculty mentors and a group that includes students from the first, second, and third year in our professional program. Fourth-year students are on rotation. The faculty mentors and all students meet each week to discuss the patients and the responsibilities we collectively need to take regarding any real or potential problems. All of us are responsible for all patients. Students mentor students and faculty mentor students. These activities include writing letters to physicians (with the patient's permission) to address drug-related problems. There is much work to do to continue to develop these pharmacy practice experiences, but we are on the right track in regard to exposing students to patient care and taking responsibility for drug-related problems right from the start. If students do not know something because they have not learned it yet, they can ask a more senior student, or they will be assigned to look it up and report back to the group. Not knowing is not an excuse for not taking responsibility. When students become practitioners they will not know everything. They will need to know where to look.

Finally, schools need to become as involved as possible with practice. We need to work with practitioners to develop practice sites, and we need studies to demonstrate the value of pharmacy services and continuing education. Many schools are developing (or have developed) external PharmD programs and disease management certificate programs. However, as previously mentioned, we also need to assist in the development of networks whereby these newly trained individuals can stay in contact to share successes and inquire about problems.

What State Boards of Pharmacy Can Do

Every one of us in pharmacy must critically evaluate what contribution we are making toward the incorporation of pharmaceutical care into all of pharmacy practice. We must be honest with ourselves about our responsibilities. This is what courage requires: honestly looking at ourselves. Practitioners must do this, schools of pharmacy must do this, and state boards must do this.

State boards of pharmacy exist to enforce the laws governing pharmacy practice. They exist to protect consumers, not pharmacists. There are still far too many pharmacies in this country that are either ignoring OBRA '90 or making the offer to counsel in far less than ethical ways. These actions put consumers at risk. It is not enough to say to a patient "Sign here" or "Do you have any questions?" and act as though our professional, legal, and moral obligations have been met. Patients often don't know what to ask or what they are signing. State boards know these practices exist; yet, at times, they take no action. We protect no one when this happens. Many state boards of pharmacy are understaffed, and this makes their work exceedingly difficult. But state boards must not allow unethical practices to continue. These practices hurt everyone. They lower our standards and make it difficult for the pharmacy profession to receive adequate recognition and compensation for needed services.

What State and National Pharmacy Associations Can Do

State and national pharmacy associations must continue to provide courageous leadership and quality continuing education to pharmacists. Associations must continue to showcase exemplary practitioners who have changed their practice and advanced pharmaceutical care, but they must also be honest with members and have the courage to point out behaviors that are detrimental to consumers and practitioners. State and national pharmacy associations have been reluctant to discuss the actions of many pharmacists regarding OBRA '90. Waivers of rights to counseling must become unacceptable to all who practice pharmacy. State and national pharmacy associations must become part of this dialogue. We should not avoid these issues. Ethical behavior needs to be explored and discussed openly.

State and national pharmacy associations have always taken a leadership role in providing continuing education programs. This includes providing programs at annual meetings and developing disease management programs. I challenge the associations to consider the following:

■ Short programs (1 to 2 hours) on most topics are not sufficient to produce significant change or knowledge of a topic. Consider longer programming blocks, interactive workshops, and multiple breakout sessions for enhanced learning. Lecturing to people for 1 to 2 hours without much interaction does not result in the needed problem-solving skills to render pharmaceutical care.
■ Consider that research has shown that pharmacists have differing degrees of readiness to render pharmaceutical care.[10] Continuing education programs

need to be tailored to the readiness of the practitioner. Most continuing education programs make the assumption that people are ready to take action, yet this is not the case. Some people are ready to go, while others need more information to understand concepts and overcome barriers. APhA and Auburn University are developing a Web site to assess pharmacists' readiness to render pharmaceutical care. We hope to learn stage-specific factors that either facilitate or hinder a practitioner's ability to render pharmaceutical care services. In this way, continuing education programs can be targeted to the needs of individuals at different points along a continuum. Programs are more likely to be effective in this way.

■ Consider abandoning "name" speakers who cost a lot but offer little that meets the needs of practitioners. I am tired of going to national pharmacy association meetings and listening to professional athletes and coaches "motivate" me. How many people actually go to a national pharmacy association meeting because Joe Theismann, Bubba Smith, or Bobby Knight will be speaking? Their speakers' fees could be better spent on continuing pharmacist education and professional development. These speakers are often supported by major pharmaceutical companies, but could we not convince these companies that we would much prefer their support for programming that helps pharmacists make an impact on patient adherence and outcomes? I challenge state and national pharmacy associations to ask members if they want more targeted programming to help them move forward in patient care (and in getting compensated for it) instead of an hour with John Elway telling us how he won the Super Bowl.

■ Consider using requests for proposal (RFPs) to attract speakers and quality programming. The membership and the program committee should set objectives for each continuing education program; speakers should not be setting the objectives. Publish the objectives for each needed session well in advance of the meeting and invite anyone to submit a proposal, with a budget, that describes the precise program and how it will meet the objectives. The qualifications of the individual should be part of the process. Obviously, speakers who claim they will engage attendees in problem-solving in a 1-hour lecture should not be considered; the method does not match the objective. This competitive process will increase the quality of continuing education and make it more innovative. Most important, it will more likely meet the needs of practitioners. Speakers who do not meet stated objectives may not be considered for future RFPs.

Summary

In this chapter I have discussed caring, covenants, and codes and their relationship to pharmaceutical care. I have tried to identify what we need to do to advance pharmaceutical care and make it our standard, not just our mission. It will take commitment from all involved. We must each ask what contribution we can make and whether we are doing all that we can. We must be willing to critically evaluate what we are doing to promote pharmacy and pharmaceutical care and how we may be contributing to barriers to this way of practice. I hope this chapter will stimulate introspection and discussion to move our profession forward. If this happens, patients will benefit greatly.

Questions for Reflection

1. Why has pharmaceutical care not evolved as quickly as the profession of pharmacy had hoped?
2. What does it mean that there is a need for pharmaceutical care, but not a demand? How can a demand be created?
3. What can you do right now to advance pharmaceutical care?
4. What does it mean to care?
5. Why is the word "covenant" used to describe the relationship between pharmacists and patients?
6. What is the relationship between patient autonomy and existential advocacy? How are the two different?

References

1. Hepler CD, Strand LM. Opportunities and responsibilities in pharmaceutical care. *Am J Pharm Educ.* 1989;53(winter suppl):7S–15S.
2. Noddings N. Caring and continuity in education. *Scand J Educ Res.* 1991;35(1):3–12.
3. Rogers CR. *A Way of Being.* Boston: Houghton Mifflin Co; 1980.
4. Reich WT. What care can mean for pharmaceutical ethics. *J Pharm Teach.* 1996;5(1,2):1–17.
5. Gadow S. Existential advocacy: philosophical foundation of nursing. In: Spicker SF, Gadow S, eds. *Nursing: Images and Ideals.* New York: Springer Publishing Co; 1990:79–101.
6. Buerki RA, Votterro LD. *Ethical Responsibility in Pharmacy Practice.* Madison, Wis: American Institute of the History of Pharmacy; 1994.
7. Dixon KM. The Challenge of Moral Leadership. Presented at: American Society of Health-System Pharmacists Fourth Annual Leadership Conference on Pharmacy Practice Management; October 9, 1999; Dallas, Tex.
8. Votterro LD. The 1994 code of ethics for pharmacists and pharmaceutical care. *J Pharm Teach.* 1996;5(1,2):154.
9. American Pharmaceutical Association. Code of ethics for pharmacists. Available at: http://www.aphanet.org/pharmcare/ethics.html.
10. Berger BA, Grimley D. Pharmacist readiness for rendering pharmaceutical care. *J Am Pharm Assoc.* 1997;NS37:535–42.

Chapter 2
DEVELOPING THE RELATIONSHIP

Because pharmaceutical care requires an ethical covenant with the patient, the relationship between the patient and pharmacist is, by definition, very important. This chapter explores principles for building relationships with patients and providers. The major focus initially will be on the patient–pharmacist relationship. This relationship is critical to the provision of pharmaceutical care.

Why Relationships Matter

Why should we care about building effective relationships with our patients? Hepler and Strand[1] defined pharmaceutical care as "the responsible provision of drug therapy for the purpose of achieving definite outcomes that improve a patient's quality of life" and stated that, among other criteria, "the provider [of pharmaceutical care] must be able to develop the relationships with the patient and other health care professionals needed to provide pharmaceutical care." So it seems clear that a productive relationship is needed to provide pharmaceutical care.

Moreover, according to numerous studies, patient satisfaction with the patient–provider relationship improves compliance with treatment regimens. In the psychology literature the terms *therapeutic alliance, working alliance,* and *helping alliance* have been used to describe the necessary relationship that must exist between a counselor or psychotherapist and a client for positive therapeutic change to take place. Therapeutic alliance is defined as "the observable ability of the therapist and patient to work together in a realistic, collaborative relationship based on mutual respect, liking, trust and commitment to the work of treatment."[2] Some researchers have gone so far as to say that the therapeutic alliance *is* the collaboration exhibited by the patient.[3] The quality of the alliance is a function of the extent to which the patient and therapist agree about the goals and tasks of psychotherapy. This thinking can be applied to pharmaceutical care; pharmacotherapeutic goals and outcomes and the behaviors needed to carry them out must be negotiated between pharmacist and patient if treatment has any chance of being effective. Therapeutic alliance is the best predictor of therapeutic outcomes,[4] and this seems to hold true in pharmacy as well as in psychotherapy.

To understand the importance of relationships, imagine this: You are driving down the street at 35 miles per hour and suddenly someone pulls out in front of you. You slam on your brakes to avoid hitting the other car. Fortunately, the cars don't collide and you are fine, except for being visibly upset. What emotions are you feeling right now? What do you believe most people feel (or do) when this happens? If you are like most people, in addition to slamming on your brakes, you

> **Effective communication is not a thoughtless, effortless process. It takes work, and it takes choosing your communication goals.**

probably leaned on your horn for a good while, yelled several epithets, and were very angry (we get very brave when we have a ton of steel protecting us).

Now, imagine that the same thing has occurred but that this time, when you are through ranting, you realize the person in the other car is your priest (or rabbi, minister, or good friend). Now how do you feel? You still may be very upset about the threat to your life that just occurred, but chances are you are now feeling somewhat embarrassed about your angry reaction. Why is this? Why does your reaction change when you find out it is someone you know, particularly someone who means something to you? The answer is that you have a positive relationship with that person. When a relationship exists, especially one that is built on some degree of trust and caring, several things happen: We are more forgiving, more compassionate, more understanding, less quick to judge, and less abusive in our responses. This is very important to understand in regard to your relationship with patients.

When we don't have a relationship with someone, when the other person is simply seen as an object, we're much more likely to behave in ways that are not productive. As another example, imagine that you have to return something you bought at a department store because it does not fit you. The clerk at the department store will not allow you to return the item and quotes store policy. You are frustrated and angry and display this anger toward the clerk. How much different would this scenario be if the clerk happened to be a good friend of yours? Would you be more willing to understand the store policy and be compassionate toward the clerk if he or she were your friend?

What would be some of the benefits if patients saw you as human and caring rather than as someone who simply works in the pharmacy? I believe patients would be more tolerant about waiting, more loyal, more likely to comply with their medication regimens, and more likely to provide information you need to make better therapeutic decisions—and less likely to sue if there was a mistake. In addition, pharmacists who maintain positive relationships with their patients would experience less burnout and more satisfying practices.

The fact of the matter is, human beings need relationships. We need to feel understood and cared for by others. As Basch[5] states, "For the rest of our lives, though we tend not to be aware of it, the need to communicate on some level with other human beings—that is, to make ourselves understood or understandable, and in doing so feel cared for, safe, stimulated, and appreciated—remains the prime motivator for all that we do or don't do."

Human beings also need reciprocity. If I met you for the first time today and we engaged in casual conversation, we would both want to walk away feeling good about each other afterward. That is, I want to believe you are a good person and you want to believe the same about me. When this does not occur, one or both of us become anxious. When we approach people, we desire to feel good about the relationship even if the encounter is brief. It is important to note that in health care we do not have the luxury of normal, reciprocal relationships; that is, we are there to serve the needs of patients, but they are not there to serve our needs.

A Mental Health Perspective

I will discuss relationships in the context of mental health. First, mental health is not about happiness. It is about adjusting internal tensions rather than external tensions. This means that it is far easier (and more useful) to adjust ourselves and the way we respond than to try to change or fix others. It is about the appropriate management of suffering. Life causes all of us to suffer to some degree on a daily basis. Our patients can cause us suffering through their anger, their impatience, or their sense of loss when they find out they have a chronic illness. We can cause our patients to suffer through uncaring or indifferent responses.

It is what we do with suffering that determines how healthy or effective we are and how productive our relationships are. Do we avoid it? Become numb? Do our defenses go up? Or do we allow our suffering to be instructive and assist us in solving the problems at hand? These are choices we make all the time. The question is, to what extent do we make these choices in a way that produces constructive, healthy outcomes, rather than unhealthy ones?

Mental health is about solving problems, and communication concerns itself with communicating ways to solve problems. It should be clear, however, that part of the management of problems or suffering is taking appropriate responsibility for problems. That is, healthy people don't ignore their problems or blame others for them, nor do they take responsibility for solving others' problems. They are able to stay separate from others' problems so that they are not unduly burdened or manipulated by those who *don't* want to take appropriate responsibility. By staying separate they are actually better able to listen and be compassionate.

In later chapters I will say more about healthy responses and productive relationships, focusing on the basic tenets that are described in the following paragraphs.

People behave in order to get their needs met. It is important to know this, because it may help you understand why people behave in certain ways. For example, every time a particular patient comes into your pharmacy he complains about something, because he gets attention in that way. If you understand this, you won't need to react to the complaints, only acknowledge the person. You might even be able to give this person your attention for not complaining.

Given their current level of and response to stress (change), people always use their best problem-solving strategies to get their needs met, even if these strategies are dysfunctional. In other words, people do what they know, even if it gets them in trouble. To change that, they must learn a new way of coping. Patients need to learn new ways of coping with illnesses and pharmacists need to learn new ways of coping with patients. It is my hope that this book will assist you in learning new and effective ways of managing your relationships with your patients.

Feelings are real. They are feedback about how we respond to the world. If effective relationships with others are to be built, then the others' feelings must be acknowledged in a very caring and tangible way. Feelings help us navigate, in that they tell us when we are frightened, happy, angry, hurt, and so on. They are not good or bad, right or wrong. They are simply feedback. We need this feedback, because we need to know, for example, when we are happy and when we are threatened. Healthy individuals acknowledge their own feelings and use them to learn about themselves and how they respond to the world. They learn about what situations stress them, make them feel relaxed, afraid, angry, and so on. This is important information.

When a feeling comes up, particularly if it is uncomfortable, we may avoid it or become numb to it. This response is common, but it may create problems. Consider this analogy: If you severed nerve endings in your hand and then touched a hot stove with that hand, you might end up severely burning that hand without feeling it. Like our nerve endings, feelings provide important feedback to us about who we are right now. That may change over time, but we need that feedback to decide if change is necessary. Avoiding feelings and going numb in response to certain feelings causes us to lose important information about how we respond in different situations. This can create problems for us. Moreover, our ability to respond to or accept our patients' feelings is limited by the extent to which we are willing to accept our own feelings. For feelings to be understood and to give us useful information, we must be able to bear them and see what they tell us. Decisions made without this awareness are often poor decisions.

But where do feelings come from? What causes them? As we grow, important people in our lives teach us what they consider to be important. We develop a set of values as a result. In addition, the way significant others respond to us when we have certain feelings often determines how we think about our own feelings. Finally, we develop our reactions (feelings) by watching people who were important to us as we grew up. Therefore, when we are placed in various communication contexts we assign meaning to what is said and done on the basis of these learnings (values). The meaning we assign then produces a feeling in us.

This explains why the same thing can be said to different individuals and produce entirely different affective responses. It should also teach us that others do *not* cause our feelings. Again, feelings are caused by the meanings we assign to others' communication within a given context.

A few more points about feelings. While our feelings are not under our volitional control, what we do when they come up is a choice we can make. Having a feeling does not always mean expressing the feeling. Somehow the idea of acknowledging or validating our own feelings or others' feelings gets confused with expressing a feeling. The latter is not always wise. Expressing the anger you feel could get you fired, for example. You can certainly be aware of your anger and acknowledge your right to have it, but this does not always mean expressing it. You can choose not to express anger when doing so is inappropriate.

The consistent ability to discern when it is appropriate and useful to express our feelings and when it is not distinguishes health from illness. The ability to delay gratification and practice emotional self-regulation is a hallmark of emotional intelligence, a strong predictor of success in relationships.[6]

Although patients ultimately have responsibility for their own medication-taking behavior, pharmacists may have substantial influence on this behavior. This is important to understand. We cannot make patients take their medication, nor do we manage the patient's illness. What we *can* do is to create a climate of care, concern, and trust in which patients are motivated to manage their illnesses.

Communication can be evaluated as appropriate or inappropriate only in relation to the objectives of the communicator. For example, a patient angrily tells a pharmacist, "You're just like my doctor—all he cares about is taking my money!" The pharmacist has choices about how to respond. If the pharmacist's objective is to let the patient know that he or she is tired of complaining patients, an appropriate response would be, "I am sick and tired of you people complaining about prices and how badly you're being treated. Now don't let the door hit you in the *!*! on the way out!" However, if the pharmacist is interested in letting the patient know that he or she understands the patient's frustration, the pharmacist could respond, "I know that medication can be expensive. I try to be reasonable and fair about my prices. Have I done something to make you feel that I'm trying to take advantage of you?"

Depending on the communication objective, the responses will be very different and produce different results.

> **When we don't have a relationship with someone, when the other person is simply seen as an object, we're much more likely to behave in ways that are not productive.**

Effective communication is not a thoughtless, effortless process. It takes work, and it takes *choosing* your communication goals. What are you trying to accomplish with your communication? As another example, a patient hands over a prescription and states angrily, "That's not going to take long, is it? It seems like I always have to wait forever here!" How you respond depends completely on what you are trying to accomplish with your communication. If you are trying to prove to the patient that she doesn't "always" have to wait, that communication would be very different from communication acknowledging that the patient is distressed and in a hurry and showing respect for the patient *despite* her mood or behavior. Showing respect for the patient does not necessarily mean giving her exactly what she wants (her medicine, right now), nor does it mean losing respect for yourself. The point is that what you say has consequences, and responsibilities go with it.

Unrealistic expectations can drive you crazy. A hallmark of mental health is the extent to which people use data in their environment to make effective decisions and solve problems. People use observations that are repeated over time to make effective decisions. Here's an example. Mr. Jones always comes into your pharmacy and complains that your prices are too high. You ask what specific items are too high-priced, but Mr. Jones always says, "It's everything in here!" Still, he comes in and buys various items each time. What can we conclude from this? Does it seem likely that the next time Mr. Jones comes in he will complain about your high prices? Absolutely. Why, then, is it difficult to accept that this is simply the way he is (remember, life creates suffering) and that he needs to complain to feel important? Why would we expect that he will be different next time and that he won't complain? Why, if he does complain again, is he labeled as a difficult patient? Some patients are difficult for us because uncomfortable feelings come up and we don't know what to do—so we say that the patient is the problem.

Here's another example of unrealistic expectations. I fly a lot—on an airline that has one of the worst on-time performance records in the industry, according to the *Wall Street Journal*. So why do people who know this performance record still go to the airport expecting their flight to be on time? My thinking is that the plane probably will be late, and if it's on time, we'll celebrate. Observing reality (and the airline's performance) has taught me not to book the last connecting flight out if I want to get home that day. Making these choices about how to behave is what it means to adjust internal tensions. It is easier to adjust my schedule than to try changing an entire airline, but this does not keep me from making suggestions for improvement.

Unrealistic expectations occur because we simply do not want to accept that life is unfair and that it *does* create suffering. We just have to decide what we want to do. We have the power to choose.

Summary

Effective relationships are essential in the provision of pharmaceutical care. We react differently to someone with whom we have a relationship, especially one built on trust and caring. From a mental health point of view, healthy people take responsibility for their responses to feelings and situations. They know they can choose their communication goals and their behaviors.

In the following chapters, we will explore some skills that are necessary for building trust. We will examine the role of listening and empathy in developing trusting and caring relationships with our patients. We will explore keys to more effective interpersonal relationships.

Questions for Reflection

1. What is a therapeutic alliance? What does it have to do with pharmaceutical care?
2. What are feelings? What causes them?
3. How do expectations affect relationships with patients?
4. What does mental health have to do with relationships between pharmacists and patients and between pharmacists and other health care providers?
5. What should be your communication goals for every patient encounter?

References

1. Hepler CD, Strand LM. Opportunities and responsibilities in pharmaceutical care. *Am J Pharm Educ.* 1989;53(winter suppl):7S–15S.
2. Foreman SA, Marmar CR. Therapist action that addresses initially poor therapeutic alliances in psychotherapy. *Am J Psychiatry.* 1985;142:922–6.
3. Frieswyk SH, Allen JG, Colson DB, et al. Therapeutic alliance: its place as a process and outcome variable in dynamic psychotherapy research. *J Consult Clin Psychol.* 1986;54:32–8.
4. Bordin ES. The generalizability of the psychoanalytic concept of the working alliance. *Psychother Theory Res Pract.* 1979;16:252–60.
5. Basch MF. Empathic understanding: a review of the concept and some theoretical considerations. *J Am Psychoanal Assoc.* 1983;31:101–26.
6. Goleman D. *Emotional Intelligence.* New York: Bantam Books; 1995.

Chapter 3
LISTENING AND EMPATHIC RESPONDING

Probably no other skills are more valuable in developing trust than listening and empathic responding. Trust is essential in developing a therapeutic alliance and effective therapeutic relationships. Squier[1] discussed the importance of practitioner empathy in predicting treatment adherence, noting the following: (1) Patient adherence is higher when physicians allow patients to express and dissipate their tensions and anxiety about their illness and when physicians take the time to carefully answer the patient's questions; (2) practitioners who demonstrate responsiveness to patients' feelings have patients with higher adherence rates and better satisfaction with the relationship; (3) patients who perceive their physicians as understanding and caring are more likely to carry out the treatment plan and ask for further help or advice when they need it; and (4) health care providers who encourage patients' expressions of feelings and participation in the treatment plan have patients with higher rates of adherence. These findings have important implications for pharmacy practice. Again, feeling understood strengthens the therapeutic alliance between the patient and the provider. This, in turn, improves treatment adherence.

As a health care provider, what should you be listening for from the patient? What do you need to understand? Is it the progression of the disease? Is it the presentation of symptoms? Far too often this is the only information the health care provider gathers. What is really needed is an understanding of how illnesses affect people. We need a shift from treating the disease to treating people who are ill. Even our language in health care reduces people to their illnesses. We call patients diabetics, arthritics, hypertensives, and so on. In actuality, diabetes is only part of who the individual is. Our lives are far more complex than our illnesses. If we are to be effective in helping to treat our patients' illnesses, we need to start understanding more about the individual. How does this patient interpret the illness and its treatment? For example, does the patient understand what diabetes is? Does the patient understand the treatment plan? Are there any perceived barriers to carrying out the treatment plan? Is the patient frightened? Overwhelmed? This kind of information needs to be gathered, understood, and responded to in a way that conveys caring. How do we do this?

The Listening Process

In order to get clarification and accurately see the world as the patient sees it, listening is absolutely necessary. Listening is hard work. It takes effort. Listening is an active process, while hearing is passive.

Figure 3-1 shows the process of listening. The process starts with an act of will. We must first will ourselves to listen. I must consciously say to myself, "I am going to listen." Next, we must give someone our complete and undivided attention. Often, people do not pay attention long enough to be good listeners. Attention is an essential element of listening. Attention must be given; therefore, it is a gift. Giving patients your attention is one powerful way to let them know that they are valuable. Everyone needs this. To give someone your attention takes will and effort. It is something that is consciously done. Giving attention requires that you not be distracted or interrupted and hurriedly saying to the other, "Go ahead, I'm listening. You just said…" Listening is not simply repeating the words back. Attention means that you focus your energy on the needs of this person.

Figure 3-1. The Process of Listening and Empathic Response

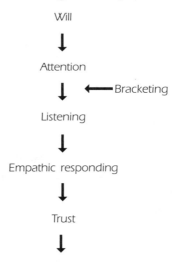

Will

↓

Attention

↓ ←——Bracketing

Listening

↓

Empathic responding

↓

Trust

↓

Further exploration of thoughts and feelings

Probably the greatest barrier to true listening is our tendency to judge or evaluate the communication, problem, or feelings of the other. Understanding is different from evaluation of rightness or wrongness, goodness or badness. To truly listen, we must temporarily give up our need to judge—give up the perspective that our frame of reference is the correct one. This is a process called bracketing.[2] It is very difficult to do. It is the giving up of prejudices, biases, or frames of reference before you listen. For example, a woman tells a man friend about an upsetting encounter she had with another friend. He thinks that this is typical of the way women respond. By definition, he has not listened, because of the judgment he has made. By lumping his friend with all women, he fails to see how she uniquely has been affected by the encounter. As a result, he fails to truly listen and be empathic.

Only through true listening can a person be empathic. The focus of true listening is not so much on the correctness of an idea that is expressed; the idea itself is subjective. The idea is not an absolute. With listening, focus shifts from ideas to feelings used to express the idea—the commitment to the idea. This is what true listening is about: Seeing the idea from the other's perspective, then feeding that back. Through the empathic response, people begin to feel understood. It is the consistency of empathic responses over time that produces trust. I will discuss this further in the section on empathy. Listening takes great courage, because in the process of truly listening to someone else's ideas or feelings without judgment, you run the risk of being changed by the ideas—of questioning your own ideas.

A common way of responding that gets in the way of listening is trying to fix a problem the other person is describing. When people present us with a problem or are having a difficult time emotionally, we often become anxious. We believe we must *do* something immediately. We want to quickly fix or minimize whatever is wrong in order to reduce our own anxiety. Usually the problem does not get solved this way, and the patient ends up feeling even less understood.

One of the primary reasons for listening and empathic responding is to help the patient feel less alone or isolated. As Carl Rogers[3] states, "For the moment, at least, the recipient finds himself or herself a connected part of the human race....If someone else knows what I am talking about, what I mean, then to this degree I am not so strange, or alien, or set apart. I make sense to another human being. So I am in touch with, even in relationship with, others. I am no longer an isolate." To put this another way, when we feel alone in a problem, hopelessness often goes with that. If no one else understands, the problem seems unsolvable. If someone can express understanding at an emotional level, then the person is not alone. If someone else can understand, then the problem must be solvable. At least, so it seems. Therefore, listening and empathic responding offer hope. The next time a patient presents a problem and you feel anxious, use that anxiety as a trigger to demonstrate your understanding, rather than trying to escape your anxiety by minimizing the problem.

Empathic Responding

Empathic responding is crucial in building an effective therapeutic alliance. The word empathy is derived from the German word *Einfuhlung*. This word means that we can actually share the experience of another. It is different from sympathy. Sympathy is feeling sorry for another. Empathy is feeling or experiencing affectively with another. It is a neutral process. This means there is no judgment or evaluation of the person or feelings involved. Sympathy is not neutral. Empathy has been defined as an objective identification with the affective state of an individual.[4]

To better understand empathy, several concepts must be understood: identification, imitation, and affective communication. Before an empathic response can be made, one must experience the affective state of the other. Empathy involves identification with the affective experience of the other. It does not involve identifying with the other person in total, nor does it mean that you have shared the same experience in actuality. It is not necessary to have experienced the loss of a loved one to experience the grief that the person standing before you is experiencing. Too often people believe that one must have had the same experience to be empathic. But this can simply get in the way, because a subjective component is now added: your experience of a similar event. This may interfere with your capacity to identify with the unique affective state of the other. Empathy takes courage, because it means you must be open to the affective experience of another. Often this experience is painful. (Of course, we should also be empathic with the joy and happiness of others.) There is a tendency to avoid the experience rather than be with the experience and be truly useful and available to the other.

Imitation is also part of the empathic process. Often, without realizing it, we imitate or mimic the facial expressions or body posture of the other, particularly when a painful experience is recounted. This is a form of identification with the affective state and signals some empathic understanding. This is affective communication. This form of communication cannot be accomplished if one is distracted or interrupted—a key reason why giving total attention is important.

The empathic process always results in the acquisition of knowledge by both parties—in coming to know one another. It does not involve like or dislike, good or bad, but is a neutral process. Behavior is not prescribed, and the other's feelings are not evaluated. You simply come to know more fully how this other person relates to a problem or a situation.

Reflecting this understanding back to the other is always transforming or growth producing. If it is not, then we are not dealing with the process of empathy. A few cautions are in order here. First, although empathic understanding is always transforming, it is not always soothing. It may, in fact, be painful at times.

This leads to my second caution about empathy. Empathy does not mean giving in or giving up. Empathy is with a person's affective state or situation, not with the person's demands. For example, a company sales representative enters a pharmacy and asks the owner to purchase some of his company's products. The owner does not carry that line of products and has no desire to start doing so. The company representative states sincerely, "This would really help me out. I'm having a tough month and could use the business. My boss is pushing me about meeting quotas. How about a small order?" The owner responds, "You sound worried. I really hope you make your quota, but I don't carry your product line and don't want to at this time." The owner responds empathically to the concern of the salesperson but does not give in to the request. It should be noted that empathy cannot be conveyed in a clichéd manner. If the owner had said what he did without sincerity or caring, his response would not be empathic.

One last distinction needs to be made. One can be empathic without responding empathically. It is possible for me to experience the internal affective state of another without responding in a manner that reflects that understanding. (Identifying with the affective state of the other means being able to sense the actual emotions the other is experiencing.) It is through the empathic response that the other feels understood. Therefore, the way we respond is very important and often difficult. Sometimes, the best empathic response is to simply listen, nod one's head, and say nothing.

Here is an example, adapted from an article in the *American Journal of Psychiatry*,[5] of how being empathic does not always lead to an empathic response. A patient is explaining to the pharmacist how she felt when she learned she had diabetes. She said, "I'm just shocked. I just don't believe it. Now I have to start using insulin. I just…," and the pharmacist interrupted with, "You just feel overwhelmed and don't quite know what you're going to do?" The patient said, rather despondently, "Yeah, I guess." She no longer wanted to talk about this situation. She paid for her medication and left the pharmacy.

What happened here? Clearly, the pharmacist accurately reflected her affective state. However, the patient did not perceive the interruption as understanding. Either she felt exposed by the pharmacist's response and was therefore uncomfortable in continuing, or she truly wanted to struggle with her experience and perceived the pharmacist's interruption as interfering. Understanding the patient's internal affective experience did not produce an empathic response. Was the pharmacist wrong in his response? The question is not one of right or wrong, but of whether the response benefited the patient. As much as we may want to, we cannot respond perfectly. We can, however, be sensitive and caring enough to observe what happens after we respond, and adjust our responses accordingly. In this case, it would have been appropriate to not push the patient any farther and to apologize for the interruption.

Health care providers sometimes express concern about the use of empathy. The concern is that being empathic will make the relationship with the patient too personal. Often, the solution is to remain aloof or emotionally distant. Gadow[6] states that "a solution to the personal/professional dichotomy can be proposed in the following way. Professional involvement is not an *alternative* to other kinds of involvement, such as emotional, esthetic, physical, or intellectual. It is a deliberate synthesis of all of these, a participation of the *entire* self, using every dimension of the person as a resource in the professional relation." In fact, anything less than this reduces the patient to an object. As stated by Rogers,[7] "To withhold one's self as a person and to deal with the other person as an object does not have a high probability of being helpful."

Dialogues

The following case demonstrates what is inappropriate (Dialogue 1) and appropriate (Dialogue 2) in terms of empathic response to a patient. I hope this chapter will help you respond to your patients in a way that communicates caring.

> **Feeling understood strengthens the therapeutic alliance between the patient and the provider. This, in turn, improves treatment adherence.**

Mrs. Allison is a regular patient in your pharmacy. She is 62 years old and was diagnosed with arthritis more than a year ago. For the past year you have worked with her in getting her arthritis under control so that the pain is manageable. You have helped her with an exercise routine and have enrolled her in a refill reminder program to help her take her nonsteroidal anti-inflammatory agent in a way that relieves her arthritis pain while minimizing the side effects. She is doing much better now than she was a year ago. She approaches the pharmacy with a distressed look on her face. She hands you a prescription for an oral agent to treat diabetes.

Dialogue 1

Mrs. Allison: I need to get this filled. (dejectedly) I feel like I'm falling apart. First my arthritis and now this.

Pharmacist: Come on now, Mrs. Allison, it can't be all that bad.

Mrs. Allison: What do you mean? It seems like ever since I turned 60, it's been one thing after another. First I find out I have arthritis, now I have diabetes. What next? I just feel like I'm falling apart.

Pharmacist: Oh, Mrs. Allison. It'll be OK. We'll get your diabetes under control. Don't worry. You're doing better with your arthritis, aren't you?

Mrs. Allison: Well, yes, but…

Pharmacist: (interrupts) Well, see, we'll lick this, too. You're getting upset over nothing. It's going to be OK.

Mrs. Allison: What do you mean over nothing? Do you have arthritis? Do you have diabetes? You don't have to take all this medicine and watch your diet and wonder what's going to happen to you next.

Pharmacist: But, Mrs. Allison, I was just trying to help.

Mrs. Allison: Just fill my prescription. I don't need this kind of help.

Discussion

Mrs. Allison is feeling dejected and overwhelmed. The pharmacist attempts to "help" her by trying to make the problems seem less overwhelming and more manageable. That is a reasonable goal, but Mrs. Allison is not ready to see this. She feels out of control and worries about what is going to happen to her next. She needs someone to listen. She needs someone who is willing to express understanding of how she feels. People often say it is hard to relate to someone like Mrs. Allison because they don't have multiple chronic conditions so they don't know what this experience is like. It is important to remember that being empathic means identifying with (or relating to) the affective component, not the experience. All of us have felt overwhelmed, even if we have not had multiple chronic illnesses. It is the feeling of being overwhelmed, out of control, or dejected that we attempt to understand and reflect back our understanding of.

Although the pharmacist may have been trying to help, Mrs. Allison certainly did not find him helpful. In situations like this we find people who are distressed, and we want to say or do the right thing to help them. Their distress or discomfort often results in our feeling anxious. This anxiety is normal, but what we do with the anxiety may help others or alienate them. If our communication attempts to relieve us of anxiety, it usually will backfire, because it is egocentric (and empathy is the opposite of egocentricity). What is needed is the ability to use the anxiety as a stimulus to be present, attentive, and caring through effective listening and empathic responding. This is generally more productive.

Dialogue 2

Mrs. Allison: I need to get this filled. (dejectedly) I feel like I'm falling apart. First my arthritis and now this.

Pharmacist: (concerned) Mrs. Allison, you sound down.

Mrs. Allison: I am. It seems like ever since I turned 60, it's been one thing after another. First I find out I have arthritis, now I have diabetes. What next? I just feel like I'm falling apart.

Pharmacist: So you're really feeling pretty overwhelmed.

Mrs. Allison: Well, sure. I do all that work to get my arthritis to stop hurting me so much, and now I find out I have diabetes. Next month they'll tell me I have high blood pressure or cancer or something.

Pharmacist: It sounds like you're worried that it's going to be one thing after another from now on.

Mrs. Allison: Wouldn't you be?

Pharmacist: I don't know, but I do want to help you manage the diabetes, just like we worked on the arthritis. We'll take things one step at a time. I don't have any reason to believe that anything else is wrong, do you?

Mrs. Allison: No, but I didn't know 2 years ago all of this would happen.

Pharmacist: This really took you by surprise.

Mrs. Allison: Yeah, it did.

Pharmacist: I'm going to go ahead and fill this prescription, and then we'll go over this medicine and how you're going to use it and find out what your doctor told you about the diabetes. OK?

Mrs. Allison: (still dejected) Sure, go ahead.

Discussion

This pharmacist was able to listen carefully to Mrs. Allison and reflect back his affective understanding of what she was feeling. He was very accurate in this reflection, as indicated by her responses.

> **One of the primary reasons for listening and empathic responding is to help the patient feel less alone or isolated.**

Although he was very empathic throughout this conversation and did not attempt to minimize the problem, Mrs. Allison was still feeling dejected.

Empathy does not cure people. It allows them to process what they are feeling, feel safe about expressing it, and gain insight into what they are feeling and why. This does not mean the feelings go away magically. We should not expect empathy to cause people to feel wonderful immediately. We can expect that it will assist people in working through the feelings so that they can move forward more rapidly than if the feelings aren't acknowledged or processed.

Summary

Listening and empathic understanding enable us to respond to others in a caring and respectful manner. Helping patients feel understood can strengthen the relationship and improve adherence to treatment regimens.

Questions for Reflection

1. Explain the relationship between listening, empathy, and problem solving.
2. What is the difference between empathy and sympathy? Construct a response to the following using first empathy and then sympathy. A patient says, "I went to the doctor today and found out I have high blood pressure. I just can't believe this is happening to me." What is the difference between your two responses?
3. A physician calls your pharmacy and says, "Mrs. Jones just called me and said you told her that the medicine I prescribed would produce about 15 side effects. I want you to stop alarming my patients!" Construct a response that promotes a relationship with the physician yet allows you to discuss side effects with patients.
4. Psychologists have said that being empathic and truly listening requires "getting lost." What do they mean by that?
5. What does it mean that giving your attention to someone is a gift?

References

1. Squier RW. A model of empathic understanding and adherence to treatment regimens in practitioner–patient relationships. *Soc Sci Med*. 1990;30:325–39.
2. Peck MS. *The Road Less Traveled*. New York: Simon and Schuster; 1978.
3. Rogers CR. *A Way of Being*. Boston: Houghton Mifflin Co; 1980:150.
4. Basch MF. Empathic understanding: a review of the concept and some theoretical considerations. *J Am Psychoanal Assoc*. 1983;31:101–26.
5. Book HE. Empathy: misconceptions and misuses in psychotherapy. *Am J Psychiatry*. 1988;145;4:420–4.
6. Gadow S. Existential advocacy: philosophical foundation of nursing. In: Spicker SF, Gadow S, eds. *Nursing: Images and Ideals*. New York: Springer Publishing Co; 1990:79–101.
7. Rogers CR. *On Becoming a Person*. Boston: Houghton Mifflin Co; 1961:47.

Chapter 4
PATIENT COUNSELING

In this chapter we will explore effective patient counseling. A patient counseling checklist (sidebar) will help you organize information you provide to patients—and the information you get *from* patients. Effective counseling is not simply providing information. Patients need information to help them adhere to treatment regimens, but the timing and organization of the message and involvement of the patient are critical in determining what the patient understands and remembers. The counseling session should be thought of as an opportunity for information *exchange*. You are the expert on drug therapy, but patients are experts on their daily routines, how they understand the illness and its treatment, and whether they anticipate any problems taking the medication as prescribed. All of these things need to be assessed if counseling is to be effective. The counseling checklist[a] is based on a review of the literature to determine how to exchange information in a way that increases the probability that the patient will comply with the treatment regimen. Each point on the checklist is discussed in this chapter. It is assumed that, before the pharmacist counsels the patient, an assessment of the appropriateness of the drug therapy will be made.

Patient Counseling Checklist

1. Pharmacist introduces self.
2. Identifies patient or patient's agent.
3. Asks if patient has time to discuss medication.
4. Explains purpose and importance of counseling session.
5. Asks patient what physician told him or her about medication and what it is treating. Asks what patient knows or understands about the disease. Uses any available patient profile information (including possible allergies).
6. Asks patient if he or she has any concerns prior to information provision.
7. Responds with appropriate empathy, listening, and attention to concerns. Uses these skills throughout counseling session.
8. Tells patient the name, indication, and route of administration of the medication.
9. Tells patient the dosage regimen.
10. Asks patient if he or she will have a problem taking the medication as prescribed.
11. Tailors medication regimen to patient's daily routine.

continued on page 40

---

[a]*Developed by Bruce A. Berger, PhD, and Bill G. Felkey, MS, Auburn University Harrison School of Pharmacy.*

Patient Counseling Checklist, continued

12. Tells patient how long it will take for the medication to show an effect.
13. Tells patient how long he or she might be on the medication.
14. Tells patient when he or she is due back for a refill (and number of refills).
15. Emphasizes benefits of the medication and supports its use before talking about side effects and barriers.
16. Discusses major side effects of the drug and whether they will go away in time. Discusses how to manage side effect and what to do if side effect does not go away and becomes intolerable.
17. Points out that additional rare (emphasizes this to patient) side effects are listed in the information sheet (to be given to patient at the end of counseling session). Encourages patient to call if he or she has any concerns about these.
18. Uses written information to support counseling where appropriate.
19. Discusses precautions (e.g., activities to avoid).
20. Discusses beneficial activities (e.g., exercise, decreased salt intake, diet, self-monitoring).
21. Discusses drug–drug, drug–food, and drug–disease interactions.
22. Discusses storage recommendations and ancillary instructions (e.g., shake well, refrigerate).
23. Explains to patient in precise terms what to do if he or she misses a dose.
24. Checks for understanding by asking patient to repeat back key information (e.g., drug name, side effects, what to do about missed doses).
25. Rechecks for any additional concerns or questions.
26. Advises patients to always check their medicine before they leave the pharmacy.
27. Uses appropriate language throughout counseling session.
28. Maintains control of counseling session.
29. Organizes information in an appropriate manner.
30. Follows up to determine how patient is doing.

Point-by-Point Discussion

1. Pharmacist introduces self.

It is important for patients to know they are talking to the pharmacist. They may be reluctant to ask questions or express concerns if they believe that the person they are talking to is a technician. Pharmacists should greet the patient, extend a hand, and state their name: "Hello, I'm James Smith, your pharmacist." This begins the relationship.

2. Identifies patient or patient's agent.

Pharmacists need to know to whom they are talking. When they are talking to the patient directly, information that is communicated is less likely to be confused or distorted than when the pharmacist is talking to the patient's agent. In third-party communication, written information becomes even more important than in communication directly with the patient. Pharmacists may need to call patients if they believe the information truly needs to be communicated directly to them.

3. Asks if patient has time to discuss medicine.

If patients do not have time to listen to the information that needs to be provided, then the information will be ineffective. For a new patient, time will be needed to establish a database so that appropriate decisions can be made in the future. If the patient does not have time for this, written information needs to be used, the patient needs to be contacted at a more convenient time, or both.

4. Explains purpose and importance of counseling session.

People listen and learn more effectively when they are given reasons for what is being asked of them. For example, patients are less likely to take tetracycline with food or dairy products if they are given a reason why these items should be avoided (decreased absorption and thus decreased effectiveness of the drug). Tell patients why the counseling session will be important from *their* perspective—what's in it for them. For new patients, explain why the information being gathered is necessary.

5. Asks patient what physician told him or her about the medication and what it is treating. Asks what patient knows or understands about the disease. Uses any available patient profile information (including possible allergies).

Generally speaking, in any effective counseling session, the patient should talk more than the health care provider. The purpose of the counseling session is to ensure that patients leave the pharmacy with knowledge about the proper use of the medication. It really doesn't matter whether the patient gets this information from the pharmacist or the physician. Pharmacists should find out what the patient already knows about the medication and condition before providing the patient with a litany of information. There is no reason for the pharmacist to go over information the patient already has mastered. Accurate information that the patient supplies should be supported and praised. Inaccurate information needs to be corrected, and information that is omitted should be added. Make sure profile information is incorporated and possible allergies are addressed (both seasonal and drug allergies).

6. Asks patient if he or she has any concerns prior to information provision.

Many patients have concerns about the medications they are about to take or the condition the physician is treating. Often, they will not vocalize these concerns unless they are asked. It is important to address these concerns immediately with as much understanding as possible. It is not appropriate or useful to tell the patient you will address the concern later in the counseling session. Until the concern is addressed, the patient will not hear other information provided. The pharmacist should make every effort to understand the concerns of the patient and treat the concerns with the attention they deserve. The patient would not have brought them up if they weren't important to him or her. If the patient has a concern that is not addressed appropriately, any information that follows will not be internalized.

7. Responds with appropriate empathy, listening, and attention to concerns. Uses these skills throughout counseling session.

These skills are absolutely essential to an effective counseling session. The literature on patient compliance identifies the relationship between patient and practitioner as a key variable in predicting compliance with treatment regimens. Patients need to see that health care providers are competent and trustworthy and care about what happens to their patients. These skills are effective tools for communicating caring.

8. Tells patient the name, indication, and route of administration of the medication.

This and the steps that follow will generally be accomplished after the pharmacist has determined that the medication is appropriate and the prescription has been filled. Telling patients the name of the medication helps them to get used to identifying their medication. This is especially important in case of an emergency (e.g., overdosage, ingestion by a child). Stating the indication reinforces the diagnosis and promotes confidence in the appropriateness of the therapy. Although the route of administration often seems obvious, experienced pharmacists have numerous documented cases of patients taking a medication by the wrong route. It should not be assumed that printing this information on the label will cover these points. Many patients cannot read, and those who *can* read often don't.

9. Tells patient the dosage regimen.

Again, many patients cannot read, so it is important that they be told the dosage regimen. Even patients who *can* read should be told, either to reinforce what the physician told them or to inform them for the first time. While a particular dosage regimen may seem straightforward or obvious, how many times a day will a patient take medication with directions to "take one tablet after meals and at bedtime"? Not everyone eats three meals a day. Patients with diabetes may eat six or seven small meals each day.

10. Asks patient if he or she will have a problem taking the medication as prescribed.

After telling the patient the dosage regimen, the pharmacist should assess whether the patient will have any problems taking the medication as prescribed. This is an important question that is seldom asked by any health care provider. Yet, research shows that the complexity of the dosage regimen can affect compliance and, hence, outcomes. Once-a-day dosing generally achieves rates of compliance of greater than 80%, compared with 40% or less for four-times-a-day dosing. This has important implications for the pharmacist. The total cost of care needs to be considered, not just the cost of the drug. Serious noncompliance as a consequence of more complex dosage regimens may result in hospitalization of the patient. Pharmacists should make every attempt to resolve problems related to the dosage regimen either through tailoring (see below) or by working with the physician to change to a less complicated dosing schedule.

11. Tailors medication regimen to patient's daily routine.

Any way in which the pharmacist can help the patient connect taking a dose of medication with a daily routine will enhance compliance. This might include identifying when the patient wakes up and goes to bed or which meals the patient eats. It should not be assumed that patients eat three meals per day. To be most effective, pharmacists should ask patients about their daily routines, rather than suggesting routines that the patient may not be comfortable with.

12. Tells patient how long it will take for the medication to show an effect.

Patients need to know how long it will take before they see an effect from the medication. Noncompliance may occur when patients believe a medication is not working. They may cease taking the medication because they were not told that the onset of action is longer than they expected, or they may take too much medication because they believe one dose did not work.

13. Tells patient how long he or she might be on the medication.

Patients need to have a reasonable expectation of how long they will be on the medication. This helps the patient to get into a mindset of compliance. It also helps eliminate unrealistic expectations. Moreover, it gives patients a chance to express concerns about the length of treatment.

14. Tells patient when he or she is due back for a refill (and number of refills).

Giving patients this information assists in planning and goal setting for the patient. Patients need to plan to comply with their medication regimens. This information can also be given in the form of a spoken contract. The pharmacist could say, "Mrs. Jones, the doctor has given you a 30-day supply. Therefore, I'll see you on June 30th. See you then?" This lets the patient know when to come back, and the patient can tell you if that will be a problem so that alternative plans can be made.

15. Emphasizes benefits of the medication and supports its use before talking about side effects (adverse effects) and barriers.

Patients need to know what benefits they will get from taking the medication. Why should they take it? Will they feel better if they do take it? A common mistake that health care providers make is to discuss barriers before exploring the benefits. It is difficult for patients to be motivated to remove barriers if they don't understand the benefits of doing so. If the patient cannot think of many benefits, say, "Here are some other benefits that other patients have mentioned to me. What do you think of those?"

Then discuss barriers and concerns. Before you try to solve these problems, ask for the patient's thoughts on overcoming the barriers. Any appropriate solutions the patient comes up with should be praised and supported. If the patient is at a loss, again, say, "Here are what other patients with diabetes [for example] have come up with to overcome these barriers. Would any of these solutions work for you?" Some patients are particularly resistant to taking medication as prescribed. Chapter 8 discusses ways of dealing with patient resistance; see Precontemplation in the section on the transtheoretical model of change.

Although patients need to know about the major side effects of the medication they will be taking, pharmacists should make every effort to support the chosen therapy and tell patients about the benefits of the treatment before they discuss side effects. This not only helps to put side effects in perspective, it helps the patient have confidence in the therapy. Remember, lack of confidence in the chosen therapy results in a higher rate of noncompliance.

16. Discusses major side effects of the drug and whether they will go away in time. Discusses how to manage side effect and what to do if side effect does not go away and becomes intolerable.

Patients need to be aware of side effects so that they know what to do if they occur and so that they do not end up going to another physician to treat a side effect. Through effective counseling, the pharmacist should put side effects in their proper perspective so that patients truly understand the extent of the risk they are taking by using the medication. Some patients may not want to know any side effects, and some will want to know all possible side effects. Generally speaking, patients know better than health care practitioners what is in their best interest. So, pharmacists must develop a flexible approach to the dissemination of information. Information leaflets are an excellent way to provide patients with additional information. Patients should be told whether the side effects will go away in time and, if so, what is a reasonable period of time. The more specific you can be, the better. Are there steps the patient can take to prevent, alleviate, or manage the side effects? What should be done if they don't go away? All of these issues need to be addressed.

17. Points out that additional rare (emphasizes this to patient) side effects are listed in the information sheet (to be given to patient at the end of counseling session). Encourages patient to call if he or she has any concerns about these.

18. Uses written information to support counseling where appropriate.

For literate patients, written information has been shown to add to spoken instruction. It gives patients something to refer to in case they forget. Written information can be used to promote more effective counseling. It can be given to patients to look over while their prescription is being filled. Patients can then ask better questions, and the pharmacist will do less talking. This has the added benefit of occupying the patient to make the waiting time more tolerable.

19. Discusses precautions (e.g., activities to avoid).

It should not be assumed that the physician has discussed precautions with the patient. Rather than assuming what the patient does or does not know, ask the patient whether the physician has discussed this subject.

20. Discusses beneficial activities (e.g., exercise, decreased salt intake, diet, self-monitoring).

The same reasoning applies here as in item 19.

21. Discusses drug–drug, drug–food, and drug–disease interactions.

Patients generally are not aware of other medications, foods, or diseases that may interfere with the drug they are taking or the condition for which they are being treated. Having this information is essential to preventing drug-related problems. For example, a patient with high blood pressure should be told to ask the pharmacist before taking any medication for coughs or colds. The patient should be told why these precautions are necessary.

22. Discusses storage recommendations and ancillary instructions (e.g., shake well, refrigerate).

Most patients still store their medications in medicine cabinets in the bathroom—probably the worst place in the house to keep medications because of heat and humidity. In addition to general storage recommendations for all medications, specific storage recommendations (e.g., refrigeration) and ancillary instructions must be made clear to the patient.

23. Explains to patient in precise terms what to do if he or she misses a dose.

Before patients leave the pharmacy, it should be clear to them what to do if they miss a dose. The instructions should be as specific as possible. Actual times of day and specific examples should be used to make this clear. The patient should then be asked, for example, "What will you do if it is 3 pm and you realize you have missed your noon dose?" The only way you can assess whether patients understand is by asking them to repeat back the information. When asked if they understand, patients usually say yes, even when they may not understand.

24. Checks for understanding by asking patient to repeat back key information (e.g., drug name, side effects, what to do about missed doses).

To fully assess whether the patient understands the dosage regimen, the pharmacist can say something like this: "Mrs. Jones, sometimes I can be a little confusing when I give out information. Just to be sure I was clear, could you tell me again how you are going to take your medication?" The same can be done concerning side effects, missed doses, storage conditions, and so on. In the interest of saving time, a fill-in-the-blank approach can be taken: "Mrs. Jones, what time will you take your first dose?" With this method, correct answers can be praised and incorrect information can simply be corrected. Praise has been shown to reinforce compliance.

25. Rechecks for any additional concerns or questions.

The counseling session may have raised additional questions or concerns. Particularly if the patient trusts the pharmacist, these questions or concerns will surface and need to be addressed before the patient leaves the pharmacy. As before, the pharmacist should ask if there are any additional questions or concerns and listen respectfully and carefully to what the patient has to say.

26. Advises patients to always check their medicine before they leave the pharmacy.

This not only helps familiarize patients with their medications but makes them partners in ensuring that any possible error is detected before the medication is ingested. The pharmacist can say, "Always check your medicine before you leave the pharmacy. If you have any questions or problems about the way it looks, please notify me. I don't intend to make any mistakes, but it's good to be cautious. You are the final check." By doing this, you are re-emphasizing that this is a partnership in which the patient also has responsibilities.

27. Uses appropriate language throughout counseling session.

This item is fairly self-explanatory. On occasion, pharmacists use language that is unnecessarily confusing (e.g., say hypertension rather than high blood pressure, or GI instead of gastrointestinal or stomach). Many patients will not say they are confused, because they do not want to appear to be stupid. Pharmacists who are sensitive to the patient's nonverbal communication may notice this confusion and say, "Have I said something that has confused or concerned you?" Any efforts that can be made to use language that is simple and understandable will promote compliance.

28. Maintains control of counseling session.

A great deal of information needs to be covered in order to counsel the patient effectively. Concerns take time to address. However, all attempts should be made to keep superfluous conversation on the part of the patient and pharmacist to a minimum. There certainly is a place for small talk in the counseling session, but it needs to be brief and simply serve the purpose of breaking the ice.

29. Organizes information in an appropriate manner.

This checklist is an attempt to organize the information in an appropriate manner. Generally speaking, the most important information should be provided at the beginning of the counseling session and then repeated at the end. In addition, support of the drug should precede discussion of side effects.

30. Follows up to determine how patient is doing.

Very few health care providers do follow-up care. Yet, abundant evidence indicates that patients do not get their refills on time and some never come back to get refills. Follow-up care is a good way to differentiate your services, let patients know you are concerned about them, and increase your refill prescription business. Moreover, patients who do not come in on time for refills of maintenance medication are at risk for further problems. Follow-up care should be flexible; some patients may not want it. Patients should be enrolled in a program of follow-up care and given options as to how they receive it. To make follow-up care the most beneficial to the patient, when possible the patient should be given reminder options: Does the patient want to receive reminders by e-mail, voice mail, fax, letter, or post card? Keep in mind that a post card reminder would not be appropriate for medications for treating sensitive conditions such as AIDS or mental illness. The more flexible you can be in providing this service, the more likely it will work.

Sample Counseling Scenario

The following sample counseling session illustrates the use of the checklist. The patient is a 21-year-old female college student who has been diagnosed as having strep throat. She has been prescribed penicillin V potassium 500 mg to be taken three times a day for 10 days with no refills.

Pharmacist: (extends hand) Hi, I'm Karen Turner, the pharmacist who filled your prescription. Are you Shelly Jackson?

Patient: Yes, I am. I sure hope this is going to help.

Pharmacist: I'll bet your throat is sore. This medicine is very effective for strep throat if taken properly. Do you have about 5 minutes for me to tell you about your medicine?

Patient: Yes, but my throat really hurts.

Pharmacist: I bet it does. I just want to make sure that you leave here and know how to use this medicine properly so your throat will stop hurting. Also, I want to let you know about some precautions while using this medicine. I will give you this information sheet when we are done. It summarizes the main points and has the pharmacy's phone number in case you have any questions.

Patient: OK.

Pharmacist: What has your doctor told you about this medicine and strep throat?

Patient: He told me that I was probably contagious and would be for at least 48 hours after using the medicine. He also said to use up all of the medicine and that I was getting penicillin.

Pharmacist: Very good. That is correct. Since you are new to this pharmacy, I need to ask if you have any allergies to penicillin that you know of.

Patient: No, I have used penicillin before. Isn't amoxicillin a kind of penicillin?

Pharmacist: Yes, it is. And you had no problems with it? No rash or anything like that?

Patient: No.

Pharmacist: Good. I need to also ask, do you use birth control pills?

Patient: No. Why would you ask that?

Pharmacist: Penicillin can reduce the effectiveness of the pill, so you would need to use another contraceptive in addition to the pill while you took this. OK, before we go any further, do you have any questions or concerns?

Patient: Well, yes, a couple of things. I've heard that strep throat can cause heart disease and that some antibiotics don't work anymore.

Pharmacist: Those are important concerns. If strep throat is not treated properly it can cause heart disease. But we are going to make sure that doesn't happen. That's why the doctor wants you to finish all of your medicine. We'll talk more about that. Also, some antibiotics don't work because they have not been taken properly. Have you had strep before?

Patient: Not that I know of.

Pharmacist: I don't anticipate any problem here. The strep that is going around does not appear to be penicillin resistant, so you will be fine.

Patient: Good.

Pharmacist: OK. The name of your medicine is penicillin V potassium 500 mg, and it is very effective for strep throat. You will be taking one tablet three times a day, equally spaced if possible. This information is on the label. (shows patient the bottle) Do you anticipate any problems taking the medicine as prescribed?

Patient: I hope not. I want to get rid of this.

Pharmacist: I bet you do. If you have any problems remembering to take the medicine, please let me know right away. I have some devices to help. Now, what time do you normally wake up and go to bed each day?

Patient: I get up around 6:30 am and go to sleep around 10:30 or 11 pm.

Pharmacist: OK. I recommend getting as much rest as you can while you are taking this medicine. Take your first tablet when you wake up. If possible, wait an hour before eating breakfast. It is best to take this medicine 1 hour before or 2 hours after eating. If you get a little stomach upset from the medicine, you can take food with it. So, take your first tablet at 6:30 am and your next tablet around 2:30 pm if possible, then your last tablet right at bedtime. How does this sound? Does this fit your day?

Patient: Well, I have class from 2 to 3 pm.

Pharmacist: It would be OK to take that tablet at either 2 pm or 3 pm. It will take 2 to 3 days before you start feeling a lot better. Remember, during this time you are also contagious. Even though you start to feel better, keep taking the medicine three times each day until it is gone. That will take 10 days. In that way you do not run the risk of heart disease, and we can be sure that the "bug" is wiped out. You can take acetaminophen (Tylenol) to help with the sore throat during that time. And again, get as much rest as possible and drink a lot of water.

Patient: OK.

Pharmacist: There are no refills on this prescription. You should be well in 10 days. As I said, penicillin V potassium is very effective for strep throat, and I am confident that you will be rid of it completely after 10 days. There are some unwanted or side effects of penicillin V potassium that I also wanted to tell you about. As I mentioned earlier, some people get a little stomach upset or diarrhea from the medicine. If this occurs, you can take it with food. If you get diarrhea and it does not subside in a few days, please give me a call. There are also some more serious reactions that people can have if they are allergic to penicillin. From what you say, you are not. However, just as a precaution, they are listed in this leaflet. If you get a rash or experience shortness of breath or wheezing while you are taking this, you should go to the emergency room. This happens rarely and should not happen to you.

Patient: Sounds scary.

Pharmacist: I know. These are just precautions. Don't overexert yourself during the next 10 days. Keep this medicine in a cool, dry place—not in the bathroom. There is too much moisture there. A pantry in the kitchen would be good.

Patient: I have a cupboard I can put it in.

Pharmacist: Would you like an extra vial that is labeled to put in your purse or backpack for your 2 or 3 pm dose?

Patient: That would be great!

Pharmacist: I want to tell you what to do just in case you miss a dose. This does happen to all of us at times. If you forget a dose and it is within 2 hours of the next dose, skip that dose and just take the next one. Don't double up on doses.

Patient: OK.

Pharmacist: Let's say that you forgot your 6:30 am dose and it is now 10:30 am. What should you do?

Patient: Well, since it is still 4 more hours till my next dose, I can take the one I forgot.

Pharmacist: Right! What if you forgot your afternoon dose and it is 9:30 pm when you remember?

Patient: Skip that dose and just take the 10:30 pm dose.

Pharmacist: Great! You got it. Now, we have covered a lot of information. Just to be sure that I wasn't confusing, can you tell me again the name of the medicine?

Patient: Penicillin V potassium 500 mg.

Pharmacist: Good. How are you going to take it?

Patient: Three times a day: an hour before I eat breakfast, at 2 or 3 pm, and at 10:30 pm. And I'm supposed to take it till it's gone—for 10 days.

Pharmacist: Very good! What do you recall about side effects?

Patient: It can cause stomach upset or diarrhea. If it does, take it with food, and if it doesn't go away, call you. If I get a rash or have breathing problems, go to the emergency room.

Pharmacist: You are doing great. And remember to get plenty of rest, drink fluids, and take acetaminophen for your throat if you need to do so. OK, one last thing: This is what your medicine looks like. (shows open vial to patient) It is always a good idea to know what your medicine looks like. For one thing, in case someone else ingests it by accident, you could describe it. Second, in case you get a refill (not likely in this case), it should always look like this or you should ask the pharmacist why it doesn't. We never intend to make a mistake, but they do occur on occasion. You are the last check.

Patient: Actually, that's good advice. My grandma takes a lot of medicine, and she should know what it looks like.

Pharmacist: I agree. Do you have any more questions or concerns at this point?

Patient: I don't think so.

Pharmacist: If you leave and something comes up, please don't hesitate to call. Our number is on the label and this information leaflet. As I said, I am Karen Turner and would be happy to help.

Patient: Thanks a lot.

Pharmacist: You are quite welcome. I hope you feel better soon. I may call you in a few days to see how you are doing, if that is OK.

Patient: Sure, that would be fine.

Pharmacist: Great. Margie will ring up your prescription. Bye.

Patient: Goodbye.

Putting the Checklist to Work

Many pharmacists are very busy in their practices and may not have the time to be as thorough as this checklist suggests. The checklist is provided as a guide to effective counseling. Time, severity of the illness, and type of medication will be major factors in determining how much or little of the checklist you use. I encourage you to be as thorough as possible to make sure that your patients leave the pharmacy knowing how to take their medications.

 Questions for Reflection

1. What does it mean to say that patient counseling involves "elicit–provide–elicit"?
2. What is the difference between counseling and providing information?
3. Why doesn't information provision predict adherence? Why is providing information prerequisite to compliance but not sufficient?
4. Why is the counseling session also called a "meeting of experts"? Define and discuss the expertise of each participant.
5. What is the difference between patient counseling and pharmaceutical care?

Chapter 5
MANAGING THE ANGRY PATIENT

Anger is part of being human. We see it expressed everywhere. Sometimes it is for good reason, sometimes not. Anger can be a very difficult emotion. Anger is referred to as an offense-taking emotion, as are hatred, disdain, and contempt. More on this concept will be presented later in the chapter.

> It is not feeling anger that causes problems for us. It is what we choose to do when we feel angry that can be either productive or nonproductive.

Both our own anger and other people's anger can create problems for us. Anger can frighten some, create more anger in others, and result in unclear thinking and impaired ability to solve problems.

There are no quick fixes in learning how to manage anger more effectively. We must first learn to understand our own anger and our responses to anger and whether these responses escalate others' anger or focus on solving problems. This chapter will explore the origins of anger and how to begin to respond to our own anger and that of our patients in ways that are more effective.

What Is Anger and What Causes It?

Anger is a feeling. It is not bad or good any more than joy or hurt or fear is bad or good. It is not feeling anger that causes problems for us. It is what we choose to do when we feel angry that can be either productive or nonproductive. Anger does not feel good (it may initially, but not in the long run) and, generally speaking, anger is not acceptable in our culture. But the feeling of anger needs to be differentiated from the inappropriate expression of anger.

Almost always, anger is a secondary emotion. That is, it occurs after some other feeling occurs. Often we feel angry after we first felt afraid or hurt. We feel angry in the face of criticism, but probably we first felt hurt. This is important to understand. The anger is a response to a threat or some form of injustice. It is used to block physical or emotional pain. If I hit my finger with a hammer, anger is a common response. If I feel slighted or hurt as a result of someone's unkind words, I may use anger to cover my hurt, since anger feels better and more powerful than hurt. So, anger blocks the feeling of being hurt or afraid or in pain at some level.

Anger also allows us to vent frustration over life's everyday difficulties and general unfairness. Although anger can be an effective way of venting, it can create problems. It can allow us to escape the core feelings that the anger is attempting to mask. Problems can arise when we suppress or repress anger or when we express it inappropriately. Let's look at each of these.

Suppressed Anger

Anger that is suppressed or repressed builds up and may eventually be let out in some type of explosion. Or, it may produce a dandy ulcer, heart disease, or other stress-related disorder. Suppressed anger is anger from the past. It is left over from past events. There are three types of suppressed anger: adult suppressed anger, cultural suppressed anger, and infantile suppressed anger.[1]

Adult suppressed anger is a result of injustices and events that have happened to us since we became old enough to take care of or defend ourselves.[1] Infantile anger, on the other hand, results from events or injustices that happened to us when we were not old enough to take care of or defend ourselves.

Cultural anger is a result of events or injustices that occur because of cultural norms or rules. This could include, for example, objectification of women by our culture so that a beautiful woman is not taken as seriously as a male counterpart.

All of these types of suppressed anger need to be dealt with, or inappropriate responses may prevail. For example, a patient's having to wait 15 minutes for a prescription may seem to be a small inconvenience, but an explosion may occur if the patient has a great deal of suppressed anger and decides to express it. Anger like this, which is not from the present moment, can be dangerous. If pharmacists see an unusually angry response from a patient, they may be dealing with suppressed anger and should consider taking appropriate actions, such as calling security personnel if necessary.

When anger is suppressed or repressed, we lose information about who we are and how we respond to the world. We lose touch with our core feelings, which are feedback about how we navigate life. Again, we need to know when we are hurt, afraid, angry, happy, and so on, and what causes these feelings, so that we can grow and mature.

Inappropriate Expression of Anger

Anger that is expressed in the form of rage, passive-aggressive behavior, or defensiveness creates problems because the real issues generally don't get addressed. Many people find it difficult to stay in a problem-solving mode when someone is yelling or raging. It is also very difficult to solve problems when people behave in passive-aggressive ways.

How Anger Comes Up

Figure 5-1 shows the process of anger. The process starts with something that stresses us physically or emotionally (a stressor). Let's use an example of a patient who always comes into the pharmacy and complains about something (we call him our PITA—pain in the...).

Figure 5-1. The Process of Anger

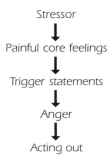

Stressor
↓
Painful core feelings
↓
Trigger statements
↓
Anger
↓
Acting out

Mr. Smith always finds something to complain about, whether it's the weather, the cost of his medicine, or how long he has to wait. Sound familiar? Many pharmacists have a patient like this. In fact, whenever that person comes in, the pharmacist usually sends the clerk or technician out to wait on him or her. Mr. Smith comes in, and the pharmacist says to the clerk, with frustration and disdain in his voice, "Oh, not him again. Go wait on him. He drives me crazy!"

What is the stressor? The stressor is Mr. Smith (or so we think—more on this later). What is the painful core feeling? It is anxiety. The pharmacist feels anxious. Why? Probably because he believes that he needs to make Mr. Smith happy. We call someone like Mr. Smith a PITA or difficult person, but the real problem is that we don't know what to do with such people. Think about this. They are very consistent in their behavior: They always come in and complain. So what? The real problem is that we often feel the need to fix whatever the "difficult person" thinks is wrong. A key to managing your own anger and that of others is being able to stay separate from the other—the ability to see that the person's complaining or anger or frustration really has nothing to do with you or who you are. The difficult person is simply mad at life, and you can't fix that.

The next part of Figure 5-1 is trigger statements. Trigger statements are things we say to ourselves (sometimes out loud) in response to the stressor and painful core feelings. In this example, they would be statements such as "Oh, not him. Why does he always have to complain?" "Why does he always have to come in when I'm working?" "This isn't right. All he ever does is complain." Notice that all of these statements express some type of injustice or expectation about how life *ought* to be. It is these internal statements that turn the painful core feeling into anger. This is important to understand. It is not what Mr. Smith says or does that creates our anger. It is our own beliefs, expectations, and values about how the world ought to be that create our anger.

Let me give you another example. I was flying from Philadelphia to Atlanta last summer when the pilot announced that we were being put into a holding pattern because of thunderstorms in the Atlanta area. The pilot said he would get back to us when we were cleared to land. To me, circling sounded much better than trying to land in a thunderstorm. But the man sitting next to me became very agitated. He asked the flight attendant when we would be able to land, and she said she didn't know. He then became more agitated and said, "Look, I've got to be at a meeting 45 minutes after we were supposed to land. It is a very important meeting and I need to be there on time!" The flight attendant told the man that there was nothing she could do and asked him to sit back and relax. He then looked at me and said angrily, "Can you believe this? Sit back and relax? Sure, it's easy for her to say. She's not going to be late for the meeting!"

What was the stressor? The plane was being delayed and he was going to be late for his meeting. What was the painful core feeling? Anxiety or fear of being reprimanded for being late. What were his trigger statements? Probably, "This isn't fair! Why does this have to happen to me?" This led to his anger and to acting it out with the flight attendant. It never occurred to this man (or to the pharmacist in the previous example) that he had a choice. For him, feeling angry and acting it out was completely warranted, appropriate, and the only response. His other option, of course, was to ask himself why he was anxious and what was the worst that could happen. If he was really working for a company that would not understand why he was late in this case, then he certainly did have reason to feel stressed.

Offense-Taking Emotions

Let's consider another way of viewing anger. What follows is a sequence that can result in an angry response or a feeling that we have been victimized. This material is based on the work of C. Terry Warner and the Arbinger Company.[2,3]

Offense-taking emotions and attitudes include anger, hatred, and contempt. To take offense is to express a judgment about the object of our anger (seeing the other as doing us wrong). We say, "He/she wronged me...treated me unfairly...talked disrespectfully to me." A judgment or accusation is made about the other and what the other has done. To accuse others is to present oneself as being harmed or upset by the other. We insist that those we accuse have caused our agitated state and that we are victimized by them. It is because of what the other has said or done that we are agitated or harmed. We claim that the other is responsible for our emotional state and for our suffering, and therefore we bear no responsibility. We are passive and are simply responding. We are a victim of the attack.

This is fundamentally dishonest—a self-deception. We are not passive. We have caused our own agitation by the judgment or meaning we assign to the event or action. We say, "You are the problem here, not me!" We say, "How can she expect compassion and understanding when she treats me like this?" We convince ourselves that the other no longer deserves compassion or caring because of how he or she treated us. We convince ourselves that the other person's disrespect now deserves ours. Yet, it is the meaning we assigned to the whole event that created the problem in the first place. If Mr. Smith becomes very angry because he does not want to wait 15 minutes for his prescription, what does that have to do with you? It has everything to do with you if you think it is your job to make Mr. Smith happy (this is impossible). It is your belief, not Mr. Smith, that produces your distress. If you believe that your job is to be caring and compassionate, then you can still do this even if Mr. Smith is very unhappy. It does not mean that you have to fill his prescription in less than 15 minutes, though.

An angry response is a choice, and as such it is often inappropriate. It is often a response to a sense of injustice, but other responses (e.g., compassion, understanding) can be more appropriate.

Appropriate Expression of Anger

With this understanding of anger, let's discuss how to appropriately manage angry patients. Let's also set a few ground rules. First, it must be understood that once you make the decision to practice pharmacy, you also make the decision to serve people. As such, you enter into a nonreciprocal relationship with your patients.[4] Essentially, when patients become angry and yell at you, you and all others who work in this professional environment do not have the right to yell back. You don't lose your right to self-respect, just your right to yell back. More on this later.

Second, for pharmacists to operate effectively as professionals, the policy that "the customer is always right" must be abolished. The customer is not always right. If the customer were always right, then every time Mr. Brown insisted he had been shorted five tablets (tablets that cost the pharmacy $3 each), the pharmacist should give Mr. Brown five tablets even if she knows for a fact that she double-counted the tablets. I have heard people in upper management who espouse the "customer is always right" policy say that they want the pharmacist to use professional discretion in Mr. Brown's case. I'm sorry, but you can't have it both ways. You either empower your pharmacists to make reasonable decisions with reasonable people, or you always give Mr. Brown his five tablets. A policy that the customer is al-

> **We need to replace "the customer is always right" with "the customer deserves respect."**

ways right is a policy that puts the pharmacist in no man's land with irrational, abusive patients. It can be disempowering and humiliating for the pharmacist.

We need to replace "the customer is always right" with "the customer deserves respect." Even if patients behave in ways that are generally not acceptable, they deserve to be treated with respect. As discussed by Reich,[5]

> Respect for humans is not based on personhood....What is sacred in human beings is not their person, but rather the impersonal in them, that is, it does not depend on what they personally accomplish in art, science, or whatever. Their sacredness is at the level where the highest things are achieved, and these things are essentially anonymous. Thus, respect for persons requires attention to the anonymous center of the individual that lies beyond any particular human characteristic.

In other words, respect for people does not depend on accomplishments and is not diminished by bad behavior. As Reich suggests later in the same article, we owe people respect because disrespecting humans disrespects that which created us. We certainly don't have to like people's bad behavior or put up with it, but their bad behavior does not give us permission to be disrespectful. However, having said this, pharmacists do not deserve to be disrespected either.

So, how can we respond to angry or abusive or disrespectful patients without being disrespectful in return? The process that is necessary involves listening, empathy, respect for others, respect for self, the ability to remain separate from others, and assertive communication.

Dialogues

Let's take a look at two different dialogues between an angry patient and a pharmacist in which the pharmacist does not use the above process. In the first dialogue, the pharmacist is aggressive. In the second, he is nonassertive. Then let's look at how the same dialogues can be more productive if the process is used.

A 45-year-old female patient enters the pharmacy and tosses a new prescription on the counter. She is obviously very agitated. You have never met her before.

Dialogue 1

Patient: Here. (tosses prescription down) That's not going to take long, is it? (angrily)

Pharmacist: Well, I've got four other patients in front of you, so it's gonna take about 20 minutes. (indifferently)

Patient: Twenty minutes! You've got to be kidding. I had a 2 pm appointment with the doctor and he didn't even see me until 3:15. Now I'm late for my next appointment. You people must think we have nothing better to do than to wait on you! Besides, all you have to do is throw a few damn pills in a bottle. What could take so long? (angrily and quite loudly)

Pharmacist: I do more than just throw a few damn pills in a bottle! Look lady, I have four other people in front of you and it's gonna take 20 minutes. Take it or leave it. It's not my fault the doctor made you late.

Patient: Just give me my prescription back. I'll take it elsewhere!

Pharmacist: Fine!

Discussion

This pharmacist was aggressive, defensive, and antagonistic. True, the patient may have been difficult to deal with, insulting, and disrespectful, but that did not give the pharmacist permission to be disrespectful in return. The pharmacist did not see this situation as an opportunity to assist the patient. Assisting the patient would not have meant that the pharmacist had to fill the prescription in 5 minutes or less. If other patients were waiting, their needs had to be considered and respected along with those of the current patient. However, the patient could have been offered other options. We will discuss these later.

Dialogue 2

Patient: Here. (tosses prescription down) That's not going to take long, is it? (angrily)

Pharmacist: Uh, well, there are four other patients waiting for their prescriptions, so it's going to take about 20 minutes.

Patient: Twenty minutes! You've got to be kidding. I had a 2 pm appointment with the doctor and he didn't even see me until 3:15. Now I'm late for my next appointment. You people must think we have nothing better to do than to wait on you! Besides, all you have to do is throw a few damn pills in a bottle. What could take so long? (angrily and quite loudly)

Pharmacist: Sorry.

Patient: Sorry? Is that the best you can do? This is pathetic. If you can't get my prescription for me in 5 minutes I'll take it elsewhere!

> **To take offense is to express a judgment about the object of our anger (seeing the other as doing us wrong).**

Pharmacist: Well, I'll do the best I can.

Patient: No, you don't understand. I want it in less than 5 minutes! What is wrong with you people?

Pharmacist: OK, I'll get it for you right away. Sorry.

Patient: Well, you ought to be sorry. Just get me my prescription!

Discussion

This pharmacist is nonassertive, and in the process of pleasing an abusive patient he fails to respect himself. This will create future problems, because the patient now knows that if she complains enough she will get what she wants. In addition, other patients who are waiting may become angry because the pharmacist put this new patient ahead of them. Certainly, if the other patients were not present this might be a viable alternative; however, the new patient should have been told, "Mrs. Smith, because you are in such a hurry, I am going to go ahead and fill your prescription first. I do want you to know that I am making an exception and may not be able to do this again in the future." Moreover, while the pharmacist should be as helpful and respectful as possible, he does not have to apologize for this patient's problems. He did not create those problems.

Dialogue 3

Patient: Here. (tosses prescription down) That's not going to take long, is it?(angrily)

Pharmacist: I have four other patients who are waiting for their prescriptions, so it will be about 20 minutes. (calmly)

Patient: Twenty minutes! You've got to be kidding. I had a 2 pm appointment with the doctor and he didn't even see me until 3:15. Now I'm late for my next appointment. You people must think we have nothing better to do than to wait on you! Besides, all you have to do is throw a few damn pills in a bottle. What could take so long? (angrily and quite loudly)

Pharmacist: It sounds like you've had a very frustrating day. It's irritating when you're busy and people don't keep their appointed times. Again, I do have four other patients in front of you, so it will take 20 minutes. I want to be sure I am accurate when I get my patients' medications for them.

Patient: This is ridiculous! What the hell is wrong with you people? You and the doctor are all alike, making me wait!

Pharmacist: (looks at prescription) Mrs. Smith, I know you're frustrated and I want to get your prescription for you as fast as I can. However, I don't want to be sworn at or yelled at. If you continue to swear and yell at me, I will ask you to leave. Now, I'd like to go ahead and get started so that you aren't delayed any more. (calmly)

Patient: Just give me my prescription. If you can't get it in 5 minutes, I'll just take it elsewhere. I don't have time to wait. (still agitated but somewhat calmer)

Pharmacist: If that's what you feel like you need to do, I understand. Is there a pharmacy you plan to go to? I can call ahead and tell them you are on the way so they can get started. Or, would you like to use the phone and call your next appointment and let them know you're running late?

Patient: I don't know. (very frustrated, but calmer) Just give me the prescription.

Pharmacist: (hands over prescription) Here you are. I hope you get to your next appointment on time.

Patient: Well, I probably won't.

Discussion

The pharmacist in this situation does not allow the patient's "bad day" to ruin his. He is able to stay separate from the patient and her problem and is therefore able to be respectful and caring to both himself and the patient. He lets the patient know that he understands her frustration, but he also sets limits by telling the patient that he does not want to be sworn at or yelled at. Although he disapproves of her behavior, he still is respectful toward her. He uses assertive communication to do this. Assertive communication respects oneself and the other.

When it seems clear to this pharmacist that nothing he will say or do is going to work with this patient, he still does not take it personally. He takes the high ground and offers to call ahead to a pharmacy of her choice or let her use the phone. This communicates his interest in helping her, even if she is difficult to be around. This is a powerful message and one that can have an unlimited positive impact on her and any other patients who may have observed what took place. The pharmacist focused on serving without losing his own self-respect.

Summary

Angry patients can give you an opportunity to demonstrate caring, respect, and civility in the face of adversity. Even if behaving in these ways does not calm the patient down, most people will think later about how respectfully they were treated (and be somewhat embarrassed by their own behavior). You have not burned any bridges, and you have not reacted in a way that gives other patients a negative impression. You can go home at the end of the day feeling good about your responses.

Questions for Reflection

1. Why is anger called a secondary emotion?
2. What causes anger?
3. What is the difference between present-moment anger and suppressed anger?
4. Why is self-deception often involved when we feel angry toward someone?
5. Why is anger an offense-taking emotion?

References

1. Lee JH. *Facing the Fire. Experiencing and Expressing Anger Appropriately.* New York: Bantam Books; 1993.
2. Warner CT. *Feelings, Self-Deception, and Change.* San Francisco, Calif: The Arbinger Co; 1999.
3. The Arbinger Institute. *Leadership and Self-Deception.* San Francisco, Calif: Berrett-Koehler Publishers, Inc; 2000.
4. Berger BA. Building effective relationships with your patients. *US Pharm.* 1998;23(Aug):52–64.
5. Reich WR. What "care" can mean for pharmaceutical ethics. *J Pharm Teach.* 1996;5:1–17.

Chapter 6
ASSERTIVENESS

Previous chapters have discussed listening and empathic responding and managing angry or difficult patients. Closely tied to listening, empathy, and managing angry patients is assertiveness. We must assert an empathic response. At times, we must also assert that we will not meet the unrealistic or inappropriate demands of others. For example, patients may ask pharmacists to provide a refill of a prescription that is not authorized. Without physician authorization, this demand cannot be met. Assertion involves standing up for personal rights and expressing thoughts, feelings, and beliefs in direct, honest, and appropriate ways that do not violate another person's rights.

> **Assertion involves standing up for personal rights and expressing thoughts, feelings, and beliefs in direct, honest, and appropriate ways that do not violate another person's rights.**

The basic message in assertion is, This is what I think, this is what I feel, this is how I see the situation. This message expresses who you are as a health professional and is said without dominating, humiliating, or degrading the other person.

Assertion involves respect, but not deference. Deference is acting in a subservient manner—as though the other person is right or better simply because the other person is older, more powerful, more experienced, or more knowledgeable or is of a different sex or race. Deference is present when people express themselves in ways that are self-effacing, appeasing, or overly apologetic.

Respect, Assertion, Rights, and Boundaries

To understand assertiveness, it is necessary to first understand and accept that human beings have rights (see Your Assertiveness Rights at the end of this chapter). They have the right to be treated fairly. They have the right to be treated with respect. They have the right to be separate from others emotionally, psychologically, and physically. This last point is very important. Each human being is separate from others. Our thoughts and feelings do not have to be in concert with those of others, even those for whom we care deeply. We are not responsible for how others feel, nor are we responsible for their actions. We are only responsible for our own feelings and actions. Assertive people take responsibility for their thoughts, feelings, and actions. They respect others' rights and do not attempt to make others accountable for their own feelings and actions. Assertive people have clear boundaries. They are clear about who they are and how they feel. They are clear about when their rights are being violated. They are also clear that many of the "shoulds" that we learned as children don't work very well for adults (they actually didn't work very well for children either). The endless list of shoulds includes "don't complain," "don't be hurtful," "don't question people and things," and "always help others." As adults, assertive people learn to question these shoulds or rules and decide what is best for themselves.

Two types of respect are involved in assertiveness: respect for oneself, that is, expressing one's needs and defending one's rights, and respect for the other person. Your communication as a pharmacist can be nonassertive, aggressive, or assertive. With regard to respect, here is how the three modes of communication are different.

Nonassertive people don't respect themselves. Nonassertive people may be dishonest, at times, because they don't believe they have the right to express their own thoughts and feelings. They can be passive-aggressive or manipulative because of their lack of respect for their own rights. Ultimately, though, nonassertive behavior often encourages the inappropriate behavior of others, because such behavior is not challenged.

Aggressive people don't respect others. They are willing to violate the rights of others in order to meet their own needs. They may be loud, interrupt others, and generally attempt to dominate conversations. They need to be right, and often they will not acknowledge the validity of differences in opinions, values, or ideas. Aggressive people often use blaming, criticism, sarcasm, threats, and name-calling in their communication with others.

Assertive people respect themselves and others. They are courageous. Assertive people use "I" statements (more on this later). They own their own feelings, thoughts, and ideas. They respect others, but they also expect to be respected. They are willing to openly and honestly communicate their feelings, opinions, and needs. They are also willing to communicate when they do not feel respected or they believe that boundaries have been violated. It is important to note that, even though assertive people believe in honest communication, they are also very aware that truth and wisdom are not the same thing. They realize that there are times when the truth may not be appropriate. An assertive person may not like the behavior of an aggressive boss but may not assert this because he or she has not yet found another job. An assertive pharmacist may realize that a patient he is dealing with is emotionally ill. He may have a very difficult time communicating in a calm, rational manner with this patient. Instead of saying to the patient, "You are too sick for me to deal with," a better response might be, "I am having a very difficult time understanding what you need right now."

Making "I" Statements

A hallmark of practicing being assertive is making "I" statements. "I" statements cause us to take responsibility for our feelings, ideas, and needs. "I" statements often force us to "look inside" and decide what the issues are. Why are we upset with the other? What do we want to happen? What solutions are we willing to suggest? Again, making "I" statements means being responsible for oneself. It means coming to the realization that we cannot change other people's behaviors. We can only change our response and communicate what we need. Caution is in order: Although this chapter strongly advocates assertive communication and "I" statements, the reader should not be fooled into believing that if people are assertive they will always get what they want and get their needs met. That is simply not true. It is not up to someone else to meet your needs. (If the other person is willing to do so, that is icing on the cake.) Obviously, the other person cannot do that if you don't make your needs known. By being assertive, you are much more likely to be respected and taken seriously and to get more of what you want.

It is important to use "I" statements to[1]
- Respond in a way that will de-escalate conflict,
- Avoid using "you" statements that will escalate conflict,
- Identify feelings,
- Identify behaviors that are causing the conflict, and
- Help individuals resolve the present conflict and prevent future conflicts.

Table 6-1 gives examples of the appropriate use of "I" statements.

Table 6-1. Use of "I" Statements

Patient Says	Inappropriate Response	Appropriate "I" Statement
You ought to be ashamed of yourself. Thirty dollars just to throw a few pills in a bottle!	People like you infuriate me! All you ever do is complain!	I want to address your concern, but I really don't want to be yelled at. It is very uncomfortable for me.
I don't have any desire to stop smoking, so quit bugging me.	It's for your own good. Don't you know that?	I don't want to bug you. I am concerned that your smoking will aggravate your high blood pressure and cause a more serious problem.
I can't believe that I have high blood pressure.	Come on now, Mrs. Smith. It's not so bad.	I can see that this came as a real surprise to you, Mrs. Smith.
You people don't care about us. All you care about is making money.	Give me a break. If you knew how much I made, you wouldn't be saying that!	I do care about my patients. I'm not sure what has happened to cause you to think that I don't.

To communicate effectively during your consultations with patients, stay in an assertive mode. Present your views in a forthright and confident fashion. People do not usually have a high level of confidence in nonassertive speakers; conversely, they are frequently offended by aggression. There are several misconceptions about assertiveness. It is sometimes mistakenly said that assertive people tend to be rude, impolite, pushy, and uncaring. A truly assertive communicator is none of these. Look at the sidebar. Can you tell which mode of responding is being used in each situation?

Situation 1

Husband gets silent instead of saying what's on his mind. Wife says, "I guess you're uncomfortable talking about what's bothering you. I think we can work that out if you tell me what's irritating you." Answer: Assertive.

Situation 2

You'd like a raise and say, "Do you think that, ah, you could see your way clear to giving me a raise?" Answer: Nonassertive.

Situation 3

You've been talking for a while with a friend on the telephone. You would like to end the conversation and you say, "I'm terribly sorry, but my supper's burning and I have to get off the phone. I hope you don't mind." Answer: Nonassertive—your supper is really not burning.

Situation 4

At a meeting, one person often interrupts you when you're speaking. You calmly say, "Excuse me, I would like to finish my statement." Answer: Assertive.

Situation 5

A blind person approaches and asks you to purchase something he's selling. You respond, "You people think that just because you're blind, people have to buy stuff from you. Well, I'm certainly not going to." Answer: Aggressive.

Situation 6

Man asks woman for a date. She has dated him once before and she is not interested in dating him again. She responds, "Oh, I'm really so busy this week that I don't think I'll have time to see you Saturday night." Answer: Nonassertive—this is not the honest reason.

Situation 7

Wife gets silent instead of saying what's on her mind. Husband says, "Here it comes, the big silent treatment. Would it kill you to spit it out just once?" Answer: Aggressive.

Types of Assertion

Before we review individual assertiveness skills, it is important to identify the types of assertive statements available to you. These types are

Simple assertion:
"I will be unable to refund your money on this item."

"I want you to take this four times a day, every day, until it is completely gone."

Empathic assertion:
"I know that this came as a complete surprise to you. There was no way to prepare for it."

"I can tell that having to take three different medicines seems overwhelming to you right now."

Confrontive assertion:
"You say you're going to take your medication as we have discussed, but I'm not sure that you're taking this seriously."

"I can see that you're a very busy person, but I really need to talk to you about your medication."

Negative feeling assertion:
"I feel really frustrated when I have trouble explaining to you how to properly take your medicine. You seem to feel that this is your wife's responsibility more than your own. I would like to try again. When you do this, I feel like I really don't want you to leave the pharmacy until I can hear some personal commitment from you."

Positive feeling assertion:
"I'm glad to see you."

"I really like it that you come in on the exact day you are scheduled for your refill."

Assertiveness Skills

Each of the following skills, when used appropriately, can help you to interact with your patients assertively. These assertiveness skills are excerpted from the book *When I Say No, I Feel Guilty.*[2]

Broken record. By using calm repetition—saying what you want over and over again—you can be persistent in your communication without having to rehearse arguments or angry feelings beforehand in order to be "up" for dealing with others.

"In my professional opinion, it is not advisable for you to drink alcohol while taking this medication." (said repeatedly)

"I cannot, in good conscience, fill this prescription as written." (again, repeatedly)

Fogging. Accepting manipulative criticism by calmly acknowledging to your critic the probability that there may be some truth in what he or she says, yet remaining your own judge of what you do.

Patient: "That's stupid. Why should I have to take it three times a day with food?"
Pharmacist: "I know this must sound confusing."

Patient: "You're just a pharmacist. My doctor told me everything I need to know."
Pharmacist: "You're right, I am a pharmacist. And I work with your doctor to make sure you know how to take your medicine properly."

Negative inquiry. Actively prompting criticism in order to use the information (if helpful) or exhaust it (if manipulative) while prompting your critic to be more assertive and less dependent on manipulative ploys.

Patient: "This is ridiculous. I can't take this four times a day."
Pharmacist: "What is it about taking this medicine four times a day that bothers you?"

"What is it that you dislike about what I've just told you?"

Workable compromise. It is practical, whenever you feel that your self-respect is not in question, to offer a workable compromise to the other person. You can always bargain for your material goals unless the compromise affects your personal feelings of self-respect. If the end goal involves a matter of your self-worth, however, there can be no compromise.

"Since this is a medicine for pain, I would be able to dispense only half of your prescription."

Sorting issues. Occasionally, in the course of an interaction, several issues will become sandwiched together. Unless these issues or messages are sorted out and dealt with separately, the individual may begin to feel confused, anxious, and guilty. Consequently, it is to the assertive individual's and the recipient's advantage to deal with these different issues separately.

> Two types of respect are involved in assertiveness: respect for oneself, that is, expressing one's needs and defending one's rights, and respect for the other person.

Patient: "I thought you were my friend. Why didn't you tell me my daughter was taking birth control pills?"
Pharmacist: "I am your friend, but I'm also a pharmacist. I need to discuss this issue with you as your pharmacist. And as a pharmacist, I owe your daughter confidentiality."

Patient: "I came all the way down here to get this filled, and now you tell me I'm too early for a refill. I do a lot of business here, you know."
Pharmacist: "I am grateful that you do so much business in this pharmacy. However, it is too early for this prescription to be refilled."

Disarming anger. Disarming anger can be an extremely useful protective technique. This technique involves an honest contract offered to another individual who is exhibiting a lot of anger and who may, in fact, be bordering on physical violence. The goal is an agreement that you will talk about whatever issue the other person wants, but only after some of the anger dissipates. Writing down an angry person's comments will often help to defuse the anger. It also serves the purpose of slowing the angry person down, because you cannot write as fast as he or she can yell. Further, when a record is being kept, a person will often choose words more cautiously.

"I am very interested in helping you with this problem. However, I get very nervous when people yell at me, and I am going to need you to talk in a normal voice to me before I can do anything for you."

"Oh! I didn't realize that a mistake could have been made. Let me get a pen and paper. I want to get all the details down about this problem."

Selective ignoring. Selective ignoring is discriminatory attending or nonattending to specific content from another individual. That is, replies are not given to unfair or abusive interaction, but only to statements that are not destructive, guilt-producing, prejudicial, or unjust.

Patient: "Hey, honey, ya got my prescription ready?"
Pharmacist: (matter-of-factly and without responding to the sexist remark) "Let me check on that, Mr. Johnson."

Patient: "These directions sure are confusing. Why don't you come over to my place and explain them to me?"
Pharmacist: "I'll be glad to explain them to you here. What confuses you?"

Your Assertiveness Rights

Becoming more assertive takes practice. It also takes committing yourself to knowing, understanding, and practicing your assertiveness rights. These rights are[2]

- The right to judge your own behavior, thoughts, and emotions, and to take upon yourself the responsibility for their initiation and any consequences.
- The right to offer no reasons or excuses to justify your behavior.
- The right to judge whether you are responsible for finding solutions to other people's problems.
- The right to change your mind.
- The right to make mistakes—and be responsible for them.
- The right to say, "I don't know."
- The right to be independent of the goodwill of others before coping with them.
- The right to be illogical in making decisions.
- The right to say, "I don't understand."
- The right to say, "I don't care."
- The right to say no without feeling guilty.

Summary

When you don't believe you have these rights, your communication will most likely be nonassertive or aggressive. Being assertive won't always get you what you want or change others' inappropriate ways of responding, but you will feel better about yourself.

Questions for Reflection

1. Why do many people confuse being assertive with being aggressive? How can you distinguish between the two?
2. Which of the following are assertive statements? Which are not? Take the statements that are not assertive and rewrite them as assertive statements. Discuss your answers with a friend.

   "This class is boring."

   "I would like to go out with you, but I am dating someone already."

   "I believe that I have worked hard and deserve a raise."

   "You people think that all we have to do is sit around and wait until you get our prescriptions filled!"

   "I am offended by those remarks and would like you to stop."

   "I really like that shirt on you. It makes your eyes look bluer."

   "Mrs. Jones, I really need you to take this medicine every day to get your blood pressure under control."

3. Why do some people have a difficult time being assertive?
4. In what ways do you need to be more assertive? Discuss one or two situations in which you could have been more assertive but were not. What would you have needed to do to be more assertive? What held you back?
5. Discuss the following statement: "Being assertive means getting more of what you want."

References

1. Ohio Commission on Dispute Resolution & Conflict Management. Rethinking "I" statements. September 2000. Available at: http://www.state.oh.us/cdr/schools/contentpages/Istate21.htm. Accessed June 16, 2002.
2. Smith MJ. *When I Say No, I Feel Guilty.* New York: Bantam Books; 1975.

Chapter 7
CONFLICT MANAGEMENT

Life is a series of problems or conflicts to be solved or avoided. Some people see problems as opportunities for growth. Others see problems as burdensome and feel incapable of solving them. When confronted with a problem, do you want to moan about it, avoid it, or solve it? The psychologist Carl Jung said that neurosis is always a substitute for legitimate suffering. What he meant is that whenever we try to avoid the legitimate suffering that life causes, we create even more suffering for ourselves. In addition to the fact that the problem or conflict does not go away, we often have feelings of inadequacy or cowardice as a result of the avoidance.

In *The Road Less Traveled*, Scott Peck states:[1]

What makes life difficult is that the process of confronting and solving problems is a painful one. Problems, depending upon their nature, evoke in us frustration or grief or sadness or loneliness or guilt or regret or anger or fear or anxiety or anguish or despair. These are uncomfortable feelings, often very uncomfortable, often as painful as any kind of physical pain. Indeed, it is *because* of the pain that events or conflicts engender in us that we call them problems. And life poses an endless series of problems. Life is always difficult and is full of pain as well as joy.

Often, the joy we experience in life results from solving problems, because of the opportunity to learn new ways of doing things and new things about ourselves. It is inevitable that some of the interactions we have with others will result in conflicts or problems. We bring so many different beliefs, values, and ideas about how the world ought to be to our relationships that conflict is likely to arise. Unfortunately, too many people believe that this is a bad thing because it feels uncomfortable. In reality, it is an opportunity to learn and grow.

Life is not about having a specific kind of relationship with someone. It is about being courageous enough to allow life's flow to take you to different places, regardless of the outcome, and to learn as much as you can about who you are (both the good and the painful), regard-

> **Conflicts have the potential to stimulate creative thinking, provide feedback, and serve as a catalyst. We can view conflict as an opportunity for problem solving.**

less of the kind of relationships that unfold. The real tragedy of mental illness and dysfunction is that in living life as often vigilantly afraid creatures, we become defensive, rigid, and closed off to our experiences. We can become fully who we are only when we avail ourselves of all that comes from our experiences; otherwise we drop back into defenses, rules, and rigidity. Real courage is being totally available to our experiences, even when they produce suffering.

Conflicts have the potential to stimulate creative thinking, provide feedback, and serve as a catalyst. We can view conflict as an opportunity for problem solving. As Peck puts it,[1]

It is in this whole process of meeting and solving problems that life has its meaning. Problems are the cutting edge that distinguishes between success and failure. Problems call forth our courage and our wisdom; indeed, they create our courage and our wisdom. It is only because of problems that we grow mentally and spiritually. When we desire to encourage the growth of the human spirit, we challenge and encourage the human capacity to solve problems, just as in school we deliberately set problems for our children to solve. It is through the pain of confronting and resolving problems that we learn. As Benjamin Franklin said, "Those things that hurt, instruct." It is for this reason that wise people learn not to dread but actually to welcome problems and actually to welcome the pain of problems.

Most of us are not so wise. Fearing the pain involved, almost all of us, to a greater or lesser degree, attempt to avoid problems. We procrastinate, hoping that they will go away. We ignore them, forget them, pretend they do not exist. We even take drugs to assist us in ignoring them, so that by deadening ourselves to the pain we can forget the problems that cause the pain. We attempt to skirt around problems rather than meet them head on. We attempt to get out of them rather than suffer through them.

Peck says that conflict or problems actually create our courage and wisdom. Without conflict or problems, there would be no courage or wisdom.

The most important predictor of patient compliance with treatment regimens is the patient's perception of the health care provider—you, the pharmacist—as caring and an advocate. Yet it is inevitable that some form of conflict or problem will arise as you work with your patients. It is what you do with conflicts or problems that will make a difference in your relationship with patients. This chapter will provide you with skills for handling conflict.

Causes of Conflict

Some of the causes of conflict are described in the following paragraphs.

Lack of awareness. Awareness involves willingness to know, as well as knowing. Someone can try to make you aware of a fact or problem, but you can choose to ignore or avoid it. If a patient is not aware of how to take a medication properly, a conflict may arise when the medication does not work properly or causes harm.

Incompatible goals. When conflict arises it is almost always because one party believes achievement of his or her goals is being threatened. The threat can be true or perceived. For example, a patient may have a goal of getting his medicine very quickly, while the pharmacist's goal may be accuracy and providing the patient with important information about his illness and drug therapy.

Scarce resources. Parties in a conflict sometimes find themselves competing for resources (rewards)—whether tangible (a raise or promotion) or intangible (respect, power, trust). As a pharmacy example, drug information is a scarce resource for patients, but the time to provide that information is a scarce resource for pharmacists.

Dependence. Conflict occurs between two parties who cannot function independently. Both parties need to be aware of the extent to which they need each other. Pharmacists need technicians to perform technical tasks so that the pharmacists can provide services to their patients that technicians are not qualified to perform. When we depend on people, conflicts may arise because those people don't do things exactly the way we think they should be done.

Values. People have different values. Because of the way these values are learned in childhood, people often see values as absolute "rights" and "wrongs" rather than beliefs that may or may not work for them. When we are confronted with an opposing value or belief, conflict occurs. Opposing values, beliefs, or ideas call our beliefs into question. This makes us uncomfortable, because the possibility then exists that we have spent a substantial portion of our life believing something that may not have been true. It is unfortunate that most people do not see this as an opportunity to question their own learning or to learn new truths. Many people see conflict as an opportunity to defend their beliefs, even if the beliefs really don't work. People simply resist change.

Overcoming Resistance to Change

Some strategies that help in overcoming resistance to change include the following:[2]

Education. Education helps to provide information that may be lacking and to clear up inaccurate perceptions about a change. Counseling patients about the proper use of their medications may avoid misconceptions and improper use.

Communication. Persons adjusting to change need support and encouragement. Active listening and empathy will offer the needed support to persons having difficulty accepting change. Patients having a hard time accepting a chronic illness certainly need this kind of support and encouragement.

Participation. The change process goes much more smoothly when the persons involved are included in making decisions about the change. It makes a great deal of sense to involve patients in decisions that affect their health and lives.

Problem solving. The use of problem-solving skills can help the persons involved to accept and approve a desired change. It is important to understand that when we avoid a conflict or a problem three things happen, and all of them impede growth: We still have the problem we originally had. We create a new problem, in that we now have to deny the existence of the problem in order to not feel defeated by it; we are thereby distorting reality. Finally, and probably most important, we invalidate ourselves. We know that we have avoided a problem, it does not feel good, and we have impeded our growth.

The Language of Problem Solving

People in conflict engage in a specific type of communication or language. The language of conflict focuses on the person: It attacks the person. People in conflict make statements like "You make me angry!" "You're too sensitive!" "If it weren't for you..." "You always do that!" By the way, most people respond to this last statement with "I *don't* always do that. Name three times when I've done that!" Then both people are off and running into an argument and forget what the point was in the first place. The problem does not get solved. Now we have a new problem. Both people are either hurt or angry.

The language of problem solving focuses on the problem: It attacks the problem. The language of problem solving expresses a desire for a solution that is mutually acceptable and achieves

> There is really only one type of win–win strategy: problem solving.

both parties' goals. Open, honest feelings, facts, and opinions are expressed by both parties. The parties share responsibility to ask questions and get clarification on the issues. Feedback is important in getting clarification and accurately defining the problem.

Rules for Feedback

Some general rules for providing feedback follow:[3]

1. Be descriptive rather than judgmental. Descriptive statements provide material useful in problem solving. "Mrs. Jones, I noticed your refill was supposed to occur 7 days ago. Has your regimen changed?"
2. Be specific rather than general. Feedback is more effective when specific incidents and behavior are described. "I like it when you come in on time for your refills."
3. Deal with things that *can* be changed. The purpose of feedback is to help the receiver; therefore, feedback must focus on things the receiver can control. "I believe I have a number of ways to help you remember to take your medication. Would you like to hear about some?"
4. Give feedback when it is desired—when someone is willing to listen. Effective feedback requires effort on the part of both the giver and the receiver. If the receiver does not desire the information, the feedback should be given at a later time.
5. Consider the motives for giving and receiving feedback. For the feedback process to be productive, the receiver should be genuinely concerned with receiving feedback, and the sender should be legitimately interested in helping the receiver gain insight into his or her behavior. "I see that you are concerned about your blood pressure."
6. Give feedback at the time the behavior takes place, unless the receiver is unable to deal with it at that time. Feedback is most appropriately given immediately after the behavior. This allows the receiver to check the feedback against his or her perception and make a judgment about changing the behavior.
7. Give feedback when its accuracy can be checked with others. It may be useful to give feedback when others are present, especially when the feedback may not be accepted by the receiver. When others are present, they can confirm the perceptions of the giver and demonstrate their accuracy to the receiver.

Strategies for Managing Conflict

Now let's discuss specific conflict management strategies. These strategies can be divided into three categories: win–lose strategies, lose–lose strategies, and win–win strategies. First, we'll look at strategies that *don't* work—that don't solve problems. It is important to understand why win–lose and lose–lose strategies don't work so that you can focus on the win–win strategies that do work.

Win–lose strategies. These have a winner and a loser. There are three types of win–lose strategies: competing, accommodating, and dominating. In all of them, the participants believe that in a conflict someone is going to win and someone must therefore lose. And at least one of the participants knows that "By God, it's not going to be me that loses!"

Competing is characterized by a high desire to satisfy one's own concerns and a low desire to satisfy the concerns of the other party involved in the conflict. The competing strategy focuses on the person and not on the issues of the conflict or problem. Often, one's authority is used to win one's own way, which leads to one party being satisfied at the expense of the other.

An example of competing might take place when a patient cannot tolerate the side effects of a new medication and returns it to the pharmacy. The pharmacist can either let the patient return it, or tell the patient that the law states that prescriptions cannot be returned. A pharmacist would be using the competing strategy if he or she argues the law. The pharmacist would win because of not having to "eat" the medication cost, and the patient would lose.

Accommodating is characterized by a low desire to satisfy one's own concerns and a high desire to satisfy the concerns of the other party in a conflict. A person who uses this strategy would feel the need to preserve the harmonious relationship at all costs. He or she would have a desire to be accepted by others, to the point of giving in to the other's desires when they are in conflict with his or her own desires. A person who uses this strategy sees confrontation as a destructive and painful process. People who are high accommodators generally have low self-esteem. They don't think they have the right to their beliefs, ideas, or values. They also think they are responsible for how others feel. They take too much responsibility.

This is a good place to talk briefly about responsibility. One of the most difficult decisions that we all have to make concerns what we are responsible for. For example, if a patient is angry about waiting, are we responsible for making her happy or putting her needs in front of those of other patients who are not complaining? Are we responsible for solving other people's problems for them? Will this help them? The answer to these questions is complex. You must first ask yourself if you are affected by the problem and in what way. Do you have to do something about the problem, and will your action resolve the problem or create a new problem that is greater than the one you were trying to resolve?

An example of accommodating might occur when a patient comes into the pharmacy and walks to the front of the line, insisting that his or her prescription be filled *now*. The pharmacist goes ahead and fills the prescription, giving in to the patient's anger without regard to the other patients. Now, several patients become angry because their prescriptions are delayed. In essence, the pharmacist has replaced one problem with another.

Dominating is characterized by a low level of cooperativeness and a high level of aggression. Personal attacks are on others, not on the issues at hand. The person who uses this strategy is driven by a need to be in control or to control the behavior of others. He or she uses power or threats to win.

An example of a dominating strategy occurs when a technician calls in sick. The technician on duty has already worked 7 hours and is to get off work in 1 hour. The manager tells this technician that he will have to work until closing (4 hours beyond his scheduled time). The technician becomes upset because he has a date planned. Rather than appealing to the technician with some sense of understanding, the manager calls the technician unprofessional and tells him that if he doesn't work until closing he shouldn't count on any favors from the manager in the future.

Lose–lose strategies. These strategies result in both parties losing. There are two types of lose–lose strategies: avoidance and compromise.

Avoidance is characterized by a low level of cooperativeness and a low level of assertiveness. Conflict is seen as a useless and punishing experience. Avoidance means removing oneself from the conflict both mentally (emotionally) and physically—sidestepping the disagreement and tension.

An example of avoidance would be the following: Mrs. Smith, a wealthy, retired woman is generally in a bad mood when she comes into the pharmacy. She has been known to use foul language when she is not waited on immediately. Because the pharmacist dislikes confronting her (or even greeting her), he always sends a technician out to talk to Mrs. Smith. During this time, the pharmacist acts busy or preoccupied, never making eye contact with Mrs. Smith.

Compromise is a widely used strategy that is characterized by a moderate desire to satisfy one's own concerns and a moderate desire to satisfy the concerns of the other party. Unfortunately, neither party is completely satisfied with the outcome. A solution is chosen (often hastily) that is not the best, most effective one. There is no direct confrontation about the issues and goals. Most people do not think of a compromise as a lose–lose proposition.

If compromise is a lose–lose strategy, why do people use it so often? And why do people feel such urgency about coming up with a solution right away? Basically, people avoid pain and the hard work of coming up with a solution that is acceptable to all parties. To do this, questions have to be asked and feelings have to be explored in order to find out what is important to others. This takes hard work, objectivity, and risking. The risking occurs because, when you really ask someone about what he or she wants and why, it may change you. And even though that change might be for the better, we often don't like to change.

An example of a compromise would be the following: A married couple can afford to either go out to dinner or go to a movie. Both partners enjoy both activities. She wants to go out to dinner and have seafood. He likes going out to dinner but hates seafood. He suggests going to the new Woody Allen movie in town. She likes movies but hates Woody Allen. They compromise. He agrees to go to a seafood restaurant with her this week if she will go to the Woody Allen movie with him next week.

Rather than finding a restaurant that both like and a movie they both like, they "put their love to the compromise test." He'll sit in the restaurant and hate it this week, and she'll go to the Woody Allen movie and hate it next week. Remember, though: If both like seafood and both like Woody Allen, but they cannot afford to do both each week, then the above compromise is win–win.

Win–win strategy. Now that we've talked about the strategies that do not work, we'll talk about the strategy where both parties win. There is really only one type of win–win strategy: problem solving.

Steps in Problem Solving
Problem solving is characterized by both parties agreeing to an outcome that is acceptable. There are five steps in the problem-solving process.

1. **Identify the problem.** It is important not only to identify the exact problem and its nature but also to identify who "owns" the problem—who has responsibility for the problem. We are not responsible for solving other people's problems. Pharmacists have an obligation to advise patients on how to take their medications and other health-related matters. But what do you do when your best efforts are not listened to? What do you do when a patient consistently does not take your advice?
2. **Identify all possible solutions.** This may require brainstorming with others. The more solutions that are generated, the better is the chance of determining the best solution to the problem. In brainstorming, multiple solutions to a problem may exist and are sought, parties understand that important decisions or solutions may take time, and all possible ideas must be expressed. Brainstorming allows a group of two or more individuals to come up with many possible solutions to a problem. The sidebar on page 80 presents some basic rules for brainstorming.
3. **Decide which solution is the best.** After all the solutions have been identified, choose the solution that is best for the problem at hand. Does this solution appeal to all parties involved?

Rules for Brainstorming

1. The individuals involved define the problem.
2. A pleasant, relaxed atmosphere is maintained.
3. All individuals involved throw out as many ideas as they can think of.
4. Ideas may not be criticized or ignored.
5. All ideas are recorded to avoid any idea being overlooked or forgotten.
6. The participants strive for quantity at this point, not quality.
7. The participants are free to seek combinations or improvements of ideas.

4. **Determine how to implement the solution.** After the solution has been chosen, decide on a plan of action for carrying out the solution. This will vary depending on the type of problem.
5. **Assess the outcome of your solution.** Was it a win–win solution? Were both parties satisfied with the outcome? Was there something about this problem that could have been prevented in the first place?

These steps are sequential, but some of the steps may overlap or be omitted, depending on your situation.

Summary

Problems and conflict are inevitable. Courage and introspection are needed to solve problems and resolve conflict. Because problems are painful, we often try to avoid them or look for quick fixes, but this rarely works. This chapter has advocated a problem-solving approach and language that focuses on attacking problems rather than people. Practicing this approach should be fruitful in both your professional and your personal life.

Questions for Reflection

1. Discuss the following statements: "Without problems or conflict there is no need for courage. In fact, problems or conflicts create our courage."
2. Why is compromise lose–lose?
3. Why should you carefully consider your motives before giving someone feedback?
4. Discuss the rules for brainstorming. Which of the rules do you believe are most frequently violated?
5. What is the relationship between brainstorming and problem solving?
6. What are the most prevalent conflict areas between patient and pharmacist? What can be done to reduce or resolve these problems?

References

1. Peck MS. *The Road Less Traveled*. New York: Simon and Schuster; 1978:16.
2. Daft RL, Steers RM. *Organizations: A Micro/Macro Approach*. Glenview, Ill: Scott, Foresman and Co; 1986:575–80.
3. Filley AC. *Interpersonal Conflict Resolution*. Glenview, Ill: Scott, Foresman and Co; 1975:41–3.

Chapter 8
HELPING PATIENTS WITH CHANGE

Change is one of the few constants in life. It is one of the few things that we can be certain will occur. Yet, most of us are not completely comfortable with change. Not only do people differ in their comfort with or tolerance for change, but for each person different kinds of changes produce different kinds of responses. As John Kenneth Galbraith once stated, when people are given a choice between changing and proving that it's not necessary, most people get busy with the proof. Given their current level of and response to stress (change), people use their best problem-solving strategies to get their needs met, even if these strategies are dysfunctional. That is, people do what they know until they learn something new. Often, when faced with change, people do things that appear to be irrational. But if we are patient and look closely, we may discover that the person is using what he or she knows to attempt to get a need met. For example, some patients may stay ill intentionally, because by doing so they get attention that they need. Knowing this may prompt the pharmacist to give the patient attention for healthy behaviors.

Managing an illness requires behavior change. For example, to manage diabetes patients must take their medicine properly, monitor their blood glucose, often change their eating habits, and get sufficient exercise. These changes, especially lifestyle changes, are not easy. In the face of such changes, people often avoid the critical choices they need to make.

Given the massive changes taking place in health care in general and pharmacy in particular, and given the changes required of patients when they have to manage an illness, this chapter on change is a long one. It will discuss emotional and behavioral responses to change, the internal processes people use to change, the stages of change that people go through, how we can assist people with change, how to assess a person's readiness for change, how to choose appropriate skills and intervention strategies to match a person's readiness to change, and finally, a process for improving patients' readiness to manage their illness.

Emotional Responses to Change
Table 8-1 lists various emotional reactions to change. Table 8-2 lists some reasons change is difficult emotionally. Let's look at each reaction, the reasons, and how we might effectively respond to these emotions and reasons. Later in the chapter we will explore in more depth how to deal with resistance to change.

Table 8-1. Emotional Reactions to Change

Fear, anxiety, and ambivalence
Anger, blaming, and scapegoating
Going numb, or avoidance
Excitement, joy, and relief
Frustration
Depression, both existential and clinical
Feeling out of control
Shame or guilt
Feeling alone in the world

Table 8-2. Reasons Change Is Difficult

Lack of confidence in ability to make the transition (Do I have the skills? Can I really do this?)
Lack of understanding (vision) of what is needed
Lack of involvement
Inability to see personal or professional benefits of the change
Thinking things are fine as they are
Wondering whether "I've done something wrong"
Thinking "I'm too old for this"

Fear, anxiety, and ambivalence. When faced with the need to change, we may become anxious or frightened. We may question our capacity to make the change and our self-efficacy relative to the change. Do we have the necessary skills? Do we know what is required of us? Is the change really going to be beneficial? Will training be available if we need it? Will others think we're stupid (or inept or clumsy) if we have difficulty at first? All of these issues can cause us to feel fearful or anxious. If these questions are not adequately answered, we feel ambivalent, and ambivalence is the primary reason people will not make a change. They don't know what to do, how to do it, or if they can do it. Ambivalence shuts people down and causes them to proceed either with great caution or not at all. When people are ambivalent, they often maintain the old behavior(s) because of familiarity.

To help someone with the process of change, these issues must be addressed. Listening and empathic responding (discussed in Chapter 3) are very important here. People's fears and concerns must be taken seriously and responded to in a respectful way. The fear or anxiety needs to be honored ("So, you are concerned that you may not have all of the resources that you need to make the necessary changes"), not obliterated. Attempting to minimize the fear ("Oh come on, it's not so bad") is not an effective way to gain trust. Comparing the person with others ("Other patients haven't had difficulties with this") is also not very effective.

> **Depending on their abilities, insights, beliefs, values, or perceptions, people respond differently to the same change.**

Anger, blaming, and scapegoating. It is not unusual for people to become angry or defensive when faced with change, particularly if they do not feel they have been involved in the process or in the decisions that have been made that will affect them directly. Therefore, when helping employees or patients deal with change, participation and feedback are essential.

As discussed in Chapter 5, anger is an emotion that is often used to mask another emotion such as fear, anxiety, or frustration. Rather than admitting that they feel afraid as a result of change, people often convert that to anger because anger feels more powerful and less "weak." What sometimes follows this angry response is blaming, scapegoating, or some form of discounting. People begin to blame someone or something, calling the change silly or unnecessary and explaining why they can't make the change or why it won't work. They may discount the importance of the change so that they don't have to do anything. After all, if the change is not important, then why should they invest in it?

The key is to understand that these kinds of responses indicate that people feel threatened and anxious about the change. Perceived threats need to be explored and understood rather than minimized. Individuals need to be respectfully confronted with statements like "From what you've said, I assume that you don't believe the change is necessary. Tell me why. I'd like your input," or "Given the problem we're having, what would you propose instead?" We can hold the person responsible for his or her statements and behavior without being punitive or shaming.

Going numb, or avoidance. One response to change is to avoid it altogether—to go numb and act as though nothing has changed: If I don't think about it, it will go away. Even though most of us would agree that this is unhealthy, it is still one way that people cope when they feel threatened.

Going numb can also mean deciding to do nothing rather than change because enough other people have made this same decision—even though all involved know that this decision may be harmful to themselves or others. For example, some pharmacists do not counsel their patients, even though they know that by doing this (nothing) they place their patients at risk. They use the fact that other pharmacists shirk this responsibility as justification for their inaction. Time and lack of reimbursement are often used as excuses for this inaction. However, time and money are surely less important than a human life.

Excitement, joy, and relief. Some patients may actually experience these emotions when they are diagnosed with an illness. For example, the patient who finds out she has diabetes may experience relief at finally knowing why she has felt so bad for so long. Knowing that the illness is controllable, she experiences relief and a sense of being in charge of her life again. For many people, change can be exciting if it clearly represents something better for them, whether that be working conditions, technology, health, or some other part of life.

Positive reactions to change should be noticed. If a patient is doing a particularly good job of managing his or her illness, this should be acknowledged ("I like that you are refilling your medicine on time and regularly monitoring your blood pressure") so that desired behaviors are repeated. It is unfortunate that too often we focus on things people do that we don't like, rather than on all the things they do that we do like. We sometimes ask ourselves why we should praise people for doing what they're supposed to be doing. The answer is quite simple. We want them to keep doing it. All of us like to be recognized for our accomplishments.

Frustration. This is a common response to change. For reasons similar to those described for anger, change can be very frustrating when people affected by the change are not involved in the process and have not been asked for feedback. Again, the reasons for the frustration need to be explored rather than minimized.

Depression, both existential and clinical. When people are faced with change, even if they can see its benefits, depression sometimes occurs. This is particularly true when people find out that they have an illness that they will have to treat for life. Many times, the chronic illness is a harsh reminder that they are not immortal or that they are growing older. The feeling that they will live forever has been quickly jerked away, and this is difficult to accept immediately. When patients begin to express this sense of loss, which is healthy, too many health care providers and others try to fix the problem rather than being emotionally available to the person with the illness. This fixing includes statements like "Cheer up. At least you know what it is" and "It's not so bad. Millions of people have diabetes (or high blood pressure or asthma or whatever), and it's treatable." These statements minimize the importance of the patient's feelings—how he or she is currently experiencing the illness. Simply listening to the patient and reflecting back your understanding is far more powerful.

A distinction needs to be made between existential depression and clinical depression. Existential means that the feeling moves the patient forward; it promotes existence. When we are faced with change, even if the change is positive, we must give up some part of how we used to be to become something new. This creates a sense of loss that can be experienced as depression. If you have ever been in a funk for a day or two and could not for the life of you explain why, chances are very good that some important change was taking place in your life. Clinical depression, on the other hand, is much more severe and prolonged. Clinical depression can result from major change in a person's life. It needs to be taken seriously by health care providers and treated by a therapist, with drug therapy, or both.

Feeling out of control. When faced with change, particularly sudden or chaotic change, people often feel out of control. To feel more in control, they revert back to old, familiar behaviors, numb out, blame someone, discount the change, or make the change. To encourage the person to make the change, it is important to understand the reasons for feeling out of control and examine ways the person might feel more in control of what is happening.

Shame or guilt. People may feel ashamed or guilty when faced with change. If the change is threatening, like a chronic illness or a change in their job description, some people believe the change is a result of past "sinful" behavior. They believe that in some way they deserve the "punishment" being inflicted on them. This is regrettable. Because these thoughts are irrational, they cannot be dealt with by reasoning. Listening and empathy are important. Staying focused on the task at hand is also vital. For example, Mrs. Jones states, "I just know I got diabetes because I ate too many sweets as a kid." The pharmacist responds, "Let's see what we can do to get your diabetes under control so that you can live a long, healthy life," rather than "Oh, Mrs. Jones, I'm sure that has nothing to do with this."

Feeling alone in the world. Even when people realize that they need to change, it can feel very lonely. People may receive help with the change, but ultimately change is most often made at the individual level. This can be frightening. Our primary fear is being alone in the world. One of the most powerful things pharmacists can do to help patients make necessary changes is to be emotionally available and reflect back their understanding. If a problem can be understood, it can be solved. This provides hope. Hope provides energy for change.

Summary of Emotional Responses

Change can be difficult. It is our emotional reaction that often determines whether a change will be embraced or avoided. Depending on their abilities, insights, beliefs, values, and perceptions, people respond differently to the same change. Each response needs to be honored and explored, even if a change must ultimately be made. For example, if an employee will need to take on new responsibilities or else be replaced, the employee's resistance to the change should be explored to determine whether assistance can be provided.

> **Managing an illness requires behavior change.**

Readiness for Change

In the first part of this chapter we discussed people's emotional reactions to change and why they have these varied reactions. Now we will examine change from the perspective of a patient's readiness to manage an illness, particularly a chronic illness. Managing an illness often requires changes in multiple behaviors. For example, patients with diabetes will need to use their medications correctly, exercise, change their diet, and monitor their blood glucose. They will not necessarily engage in each of these behaviors equally well, nor are they likely to engage in each of the behaviors with the same degree of motivation or commitment. This part of the chapter will examine a model of change and discuss how pharmacists and other health care providers can assist patients in managing their illnesses.

The Transtheoretical Model of Change

During the 1970s and 1980s, Prochaska and colleagues did an exhaustive examination of the literature on change.[1,2] They looked at why and how people change in therapy, why they do not change, and why and how they change outside of therapy. They examined change across more than 200 different psychotherapies. The objective was to develop a comprehensive model that could be used to predict how ready an individual is for change and how to intervene to assist the individual in making the change.

From this research, the transtheoretical model of change was developed. In summary, Prochaska and colleagues were able to identify 5 stages of readiness for change (Table 8-3) and 10 processes of change (Table 8-4) that individuals use to move from one stage of readiness to the next. In other words, change is not an either/or process.[3,4] People often cycle through the five stages of change (or readiness) before the change is internalized and habituated. The first three stages are cognitive. That is, people think about the change and weigh the pros and cons of making the change. They also decide whether they have the skills and resources to make the necessary changes (self-efficacy). While in each stage of readiness, people use different internal processes (Table 8-4) to move to the next stage.

It is the health care provider's task to assess the patient's readiness to manage the target behaviors and then use stage-specific skills and strategies to stimulate the internal processes used to motivate change and help the patient move to the next stage of readiness. Notice that the task is not necessarily to move the patient directly to action. It is to help the patient move to the next stage.

For example, one internal process is consciousness-raising. It is the most-used process of change. Increasing the information available to the patient can help the patient make better choices. For patients with diabetes to successfully manage their

Table 8-3. Stages of Change and Pharmacist Support

Stage	Characteristics	Skills/Interventions by Pharmacist
Precontemplation	Unaware, unwilling, too discouraged, have not tried anything, cons outweigh pros, not ready to try anything within next 6 months	Listening and empathic responding, effective questioning, identifying barriers to change, nonjudgmental approach; persuasive strategies are generally ineffective; avoid argumentation in all stages
Contemplation	Open to information, education; thinking about trying something within 6 months; low self-efficacy; high perceived temptation to stay the same	Listening and empathic responding, educational interventions, emotional support, social support, effective questioning, discussion of strategies to remove barriers, developing discrepancies
Preparation	Ready to engage in behavior(s) in the next month, have made at least one prior attempt in the past year, beginning to set goals and "psych" self up	Listening and empathy, praise for readiness to manage illness, assistance in setting goals, discussion of plan of action, identification of pitfalls, asking about support of others
Action	Taking steps; fighting "coercive forces"; engaging willpower, developing a sense of autonomy; improved self-efficacy, but may also experience guilt, failure, limits of personal freedom; very stressful stage	Listening and empathy; reinforcement of self-efficacious behavior; encouragement; continued emotional support, especially if relapse occurs; identification of reasons for relapse; confrontation may be necessary; avoid argumentation
Maintenance	Engaged in new behaviors for at least 6 months; senses that "I am becoming more like the person I want to be"; is able to more clearly identify situations and self-defeating behaviors that encourage relapse	Listening and empathy, open assessment of situations likely to produce relapse, continued use of counterconditioning and stimulus control, continued support and positive reinforcement

illness, they must first know enough about the illness and how to control it. Therefore, their understanding of the illness and its treatment must be assessed and then appropriate information must be communicated. Although education does not predict adherence, it is vital that patients assimilate *accurate* information so that they have a reasonable chance to succeed. Thus, education is an intervention that can stimulate the internal process, consciousness-raising, in the patient.

Table 8-4. Processes of Change and Most Prominent Stages

Process	Peak Stage
Social liberation: noticing that others with a similar condition in their environment are changing behaviors	Contemplation, preparation
Dramatic relief: becoming upset or emotional in response to information about the hazards of not changing	Precontemplation, contemplation
Helping relationships: the existence of meaningful or salient others who provide support for one's change efforts	Preparation, action, and maintenance
Consciousness-raising: gaining and thinking about information that is relevant to one's health maintenance behaviors	Precontemplation, contemplation
Environmental re-evaluation: recognizing the harmful effects of not taking care of oneself on the physical and social environments	Contemplation
Reinforcement management: rewarding oneself or being rewarded by others for healthy behaviors	Action, maintenance
Self-re-evaluation: cognitively evaluating one's attitudes toward healthy and unhealthy behaviors	Contemplation
Stimulus control: altering or manipulating the environment to remove cues that trigger relapses in behaviors and introducing cues to facilitate healthy behaviors	Action, maintenance
Counterconditioning: developing and engaging in new behaviors to take the place of a behavior such as overeating	Action, maintenance
Self-liberation: realizing that one is capable of successfully engaging in healthy behaviors if one chooses	Preparation

This model is very powerful, yet sometimes it presents difficulties for health care providers who have a strong need for control or believe that *they* manage the patient's illness. In reality, we cannot control, motivate, or save the patient. Nor do health care providers manage an illness. Patients manage illnesses, or they don't. What we *can* do is provide sufficient, understandable information in a caring, trusting context in which patients feel safe enough and free enough to discuss their successes and problems in managing their illnesses. In addition, we can use patient-specific skills and strategies to help patients move toward healthy behaviors. Table 8-5 contrasts the biomedical (paternalistic) model of care with a socio-behavioral model of care. The biomedical model is one in which the health care provider is in control. In the socio-behavioral model, the patient and provider are partners who negotiate care. The biomedical model works in settings such as hospitals and nursing homes. However, it does not work well at all when the patient is ambulatory and can choose whether or not to follow a treatment regimen; this is where socio-behavioral models work best. The transtheoretical model is a socio-behavioral model of care.

Table 8-5. Traditional versus Empowerment Model of Care

Biomedical Model (Paternalistic)	Socio-behavioral Model
Practitioner centered	Patient centered
Information giving	Information exchange (a meeting of experts)
Practitioner must "save" the patient	Patients must save themselves
Dictate behavior	Negotiate behavior
Compliance	Adherence
Authoritarian (parent–child) relationship	Servant
Motivate the patient	Assess the patient's motivation
Persuade, manipulate	Understand, accept
Resistance is bad	Resistance is information
Argue	Confront
Respect is expected	Mutual respect is assumed

Some Important Contrasts

Before further discussion of the stages of change, let's look at some important contrasts (Table 8-6). When people are faced with change, initially the change may seem foreign to them. This is especially true when they are told they have a chronic illness to manage. They may say, "It's not happening to me" or "It's not really that serious." In other words, they don't accept what is happening to them. Until the change or illness is internalized or integrated and becomes part of who the person is, the change is unlikely to take place. Empathy, understanding, and education assist in the process of internalization.

Ambivalence is a major reason people don't change. If they don't know what to do or how to do it, or do not believe they have the skills or resources to do what is necessary, change usually does not occur. Therefore, interventions that help people understand what is needed and the resultant benefits are often useful. In addition, dissonance is a powerful promoter of change. If people believe that staying the same will create more problems than changing, change is more likely. Dissonance stimulates self-re-evaluation. In order to change, the patient must decide that he will like himself more as a result of the changes. More on creating dissonance later.

Table 8-6. Important Contrasts

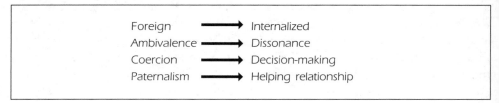

Foreign ⟶ Internalized
Ambivalence ⟶ Dissonance
Coercion ⟶ Decision-making
Paternalism ⟶ Helping relationship

People are less likely to change if they feel coerced or feel their freedom is being impinged on. People are more likely to change when they believe the decision is theirs. Good decision-making is aided by accurate, nonjudgmental information, empathic understanding, and emphasis on the benefits of making the change.

Finally, helping relationships are far more likely than paternalism (treating patients like children) to move people toward change. Helping relationships involve the patient in the decision-making, respect that this change is only part of what is occurring in the patient's life, and allow the patient to express fears, doubts, or concerns. Helping relationships stimulate self-liberation: Patients feel free to make better choices. Still, there are patients who want to be told exactly what to do and when. But even this is a choice that the patient, not the health care provider, is making.

The Stages of Change

Next we will discuss a process for assessing the patient's readiness to engage in a behavior and identifying perceived barriers to change and possible benefits of change. The stages of change and the interventions and skills to be used by the pharmacist in each stage are summarized in Table 8-3.

Precontemplation. This is the first stage of readiness. Individuals in this stage are unaware, unwilling, or too discouraged to change. For the precontemplator who is unaware, the best strategy is education. For example, people with diabetes cannot effectively manage their illness if they do not understand the illness or its treatment.

For patients who are aware but unwilling, a different approach is needed. Many smokers are aware of the dangers of smoking but continue to smoke. Here, a strategy is to ask the smoker what he or she likes about smoking. If the smoker says, "It relaxes me," a helpful response is, "It would be hard to give up something that is relaxing." This response does not put the patient on the defensive and, in fact, demonstrates nonjudgmental understanding. After asking what else the smoker likes about smoking, ask what he or she sees as the downside of smoking. Summarize all that you have heard, saying, "So, on the one hand you like smoking because... while on the other hand you see the downside of smoking as..." This is called *developing discrepancies*. Saying the pros and cons out loud creates dissonance, and dissonance creates motivation for change.

To assess just how resistant to change the patient is, the "envelope" method is recommended. Using our smoking example, you would say, "Mr. Smith, if I were to hand you an envelope, what message would have to be inside it for you to consider quitting?" Hard-core precontemplators will tell you, "There isn't any message that could get me to quit." Some patients have no intention of changing, and we cannot save them. We would simply say, "Mr. Smith, it sounds like you're not ready to quit smoking. I am concerned that your smoking increases your chances for a stroke or heart attack because of your high blood pressure, but it really is up to you whether you want to quit. If you get to the point where you are considering quitting, let me know and I will be glad to help you with some methods for doing so." On the other hand, when asked about the envelope, some patients might say, "I guess if I found out that I had early warning signs of problems." Now you can ask them to consider getting their lungs checked so they can make a better decision about whether to consider quitting.

A similar method for dealing with resistant patients uses "readiness rulers" to assess both how important the patient perceives managing the illness to be and how self-efficacious he or she feels about doing so. Readiness rulers for measuring importance would go like this: "On a scale from 1 to 7, where 1 is not at all important and 7 is extremely important, how important to you is taking your medicine properly to manage your diabetes?" Let's say that the patient answers "3." The mistake the health care provider typically makes is to say, "Why a 3 and not a 7?" This response forces patients to talk negatively about the behavior—for example, why they don't think it is important to take their medicine. A more productive response is to say, "Why a 3 and not a 1?" This elicits change talk from the patient. If the patient says "1," you know the patient is not ready, and an appropriate response would be, "It does not sound like you are ready to take your medicine as prescribed. What would have to happen for you to be ready?" After listening carefully to the patient's answer to "Why a 3 and not a 1?" it is useful to then say, "What would have to happen for you to move to a 4?" This gets the patient thinking about change, but in a small, incremental way. It helps the patient think about change and what it would take to be more committed to change, but it does so in an incremental way. Asking about a 6 or 7 at this point would be too much and could cause resistance.

For patients who are too discouraged to change, it is helpful to identify any successes they have had in past change attempts. Identifying what worked, even for a short period of time, can help the patient repeat these actions for longer periods.

Contemplation. In this stage, patients are more open to information and want to learn more. They are thinking of changing in the next 6 months. Providing objective, nonjudgmental information is very important in this stage. Noticing the patient's statements indicating a shift in his or her stage of readiness is also important. Asking the patient what he or she anticipates will be the greatest obstacles and what he or she perceives as the benefits of the change is very useful.

Preparation. The patient is getting ready to try something in the next 30 days. It is not until this stage that any action-oriented strategies are considered. Setting small goals and removing barriers to change are very important in this stage. Discussing the patient's plan for action and praising his or her readiness also are very important.

Action. This stage is critical. A great deal of effort is being made. The patient has now engaged in the behavior(s), but for less than 6 months. Often we think our work is done at this point, but it is really just beginning. Patients need to be noticed. The new behaviors need to be reinforced. "Cheerleading" and social support are essential. Unfortunately, major improvements may go unnoticed because health care providers and family can't understand why they should praise a patient for doing what he's supposed to be doing. The answer is simple. You want him to keep doing it. Statements like "Mr. Jones, I noticed that you were right on time for your blood pressure medicine this month. Way to go. I wish more of my patients took their blood pressure as seriously as you do. How have you been able to get yourself on track? I'd like to be able to tell some of my other patients" are very helpful and encouraging.

> The transtheoretical model of change helps us to understand that change is a process and that each stage of the process requires different skills and strategies for effectively helping the patient to change.

Maintenance. In this stage, the patient has been engaged in the target behavior(s) for at least 6 months. Again, noticing the positive changes is very important. Relapse prevention is a focus of this stage. At some time or another, patients may relapse. The smoker may smoke, the patient with diabetes may get off his diet, and so on. The key is to stay focused on attacking problems, not people. For example:

Pharmacist: Mrs. Jones, what happened to cause your blood glucose to go up?

Mrs. Jones: We had a rash of birthdays at work. You know, cake, ice cream, the works. I overindulged.

Pharmacist: OK, that happens now and then. Since you were doing a great job of keeping your diabetes under control, I know that you'll get back on track. What's your plan?

Mrs. Jones: Smaller piece of cake, no ice cream.

The pharmacist's communication is supportive, encouraging, and nonjudgmental.

Summary of the Transtheoretical Model

The transtheoretical model of change helps us to understand that change is a process and each stage of the process requires different skills and strategies for effectively helping the patient to change.

Motivational Interviewing

Now we will take what we have learned about change and put it all together in a process called motivational interviewing. This process will assist you in using the skills and concepts we have discussed. A step-by-step approach will help you identify the patient's readiness and understanding. In addition, you will be shown how all of this fits into patient counseling and medication history taking.

Motivational interviewing was originally developed by Miller and Rollnick[5] as a complementary process to the transtheoretical model of change. It was first targeted toward people with addictive behaviors but, with the development of brief motivational interviewing, it is now being used to assist health care providers in managing patients with other illnesses.[6] The object of motivational interviewing and brief motivational interviewing is to negotiate behavior change with a patient or client.

As developed by Miller and Rollnick,[5] motivational interviewing is a strategy for helping patients make a commitment to change. It combines Rogers's[7] client-centered approach to therapy and more directive approaches for helping people change. The basic idea behind motivational interviewing is that, for any number of reasons, patients are often ambivalent about change. They may not be aware that a change is truly needed. They may have misinterpreted the seriousness of the condition. They may understand the treatment regimen but be unable to carry it out without great difficulty. As a result, they're not sure they have what it takes to control their illness.

Ambivalence affects readiness to change and inhibits the adoption of strategies for change. Motivational interviewing starts with an assessment of the patient's readiness to change. Knowing what stage a patient is in helps the practitioner to identify strategies to promote change. For example, individuals in the precontemplation stage may not be aware that there is a problem. They need objective, nonjudgmental information. On the other hand, people in the action stage are ready for change. With these individuals, the pharmacist may want to check the accuracy of their information to ensure that their attempts to change (their coping strategies) are appropriate. These patients have made a commitment to change, so encouragement and help in defining strategies work well.

Motivational interviewing is extremely useful because it teaches the health care provider to explore the patient's understanding and concerns. It focuses on dealing with resistance and helping patients move through the stages of change.

> **People are much more highly motivated to change when discrepancies exist between current behavior and desired personal goals. Motivational interviewing attempts to create these discrepancies without making the patient feel threatened or pressured.**

Strategies for Motivational Interviewing

Motivational interviewing focuses on a menu of interview strategies and five supporting principles (sidebar, page 96) for identifying the patient's stage of change and assisting in change. The menu of strategies is modified from the work of Rollnick and colleagues.[6] A skilled provider can use the entire menu of interview strategies with a patient in no more than 5 to 15 minutes. An individual patient may require some or all of the items, depending on where the patient is in the process. Each time the patient is seen, some or all of the strategies will be used.

1. Opening strategy: Lifestyle. This strategy involves talking in general about the patient's lifestyle from the patient's own perspective. Does the patient view it as healthy or unhealthy? What does the patient like or dislike about it? Does the patient exercise? How much? Are there aspects that need to change? This opening strategy gives the pharmacist a general picture of the patient's health habits (or lack of them) and desire to change unhealthy habits or take on new behaviors.

2. A typical day. This strategy helps the pharmacist at several levels. Knowing what a typical day is like for the patient allows the pharmacist to do a better job of realistically tailoring medication regimens (or exercise or other factors) to fit the patient's daily routines. Tailoring can greatly improve treatment adherence, because patients can attach medication taking to a behavior or activity they are used to doing. Also, knowing how the patient's day is structured can help in planning. There is no point in telling a patient to monitor her blood glucose at 3 pm when that is a busy time for her each day. This strategy also helps to build rapport with the patient.

3. The good things and the less good things. This strategy helps the pharmacist continue to build rapport and allows exploration of how a patient represents his or her illness and its treatment. Patients with misconceptions about an illness or its treatment may treat the illness inappropriately. By asking patients questions such as "What does having diabetes mean to you?" the pharmacist is able to determine which beliefs are accurate and which need to be corrected. In discussing the good things and the less good things, the pharmacist can also ask patients about what they perceive as barriers and facilitators to treating their illness.

All of this gives the pharmacist the opportunity to listen to the patient and demonstrate understanding by responding empathically. Identifying barriers to and facilitators of behavior change also allows the pharmacist to more accurately determine the patient's stage of readiness. Barriers to change are much more prominent in the earlier stages. Finally, knowing the good things and the less good things gives the pharmacist the opportunity to develop discrepancies between old, unwanted behaviors and new, desired behaviors. This is an effective skill for moving patients forward (more on this later).

4. Providing information. This strategy is really aimed at *exchanging* further information. This is where the patient counseling checklist (Chapter 4) fits into the process. First, the pharmacist should ask if the patient wants additional information about the illness and its treatment (or about smoking cessation or some other topic). If the patient is not ready for more information, it is wise to note this and provide only a leaflet. It does not make sense to try to tell patients more when they are not ready to hear it. If the patient is ready for additional information, it should be provided in an unbiased, nonjudgmental manner. The information provided should assist patients in taking their medications appropriately. Patients should leave the pharmacy with a clear understanding of what to expect and what to do if the expected doesn't occur. (For a thorough discussion of the kind of information to be provided, see Chapter 4.)

5. The future and the present. This strategy allows patients to discuss what they want to have happen as a result of treating the illness. Usually, any concern or dissatisfaction on the part of the patient will come out here and should be addressed in a compassionate, nonjudgmental manner.

6. Helping with decision-making. Finally, the pharmacist should assist patients in making decisions about managing their illnesses. Patients should be asked questions like "What are your thoughts now about managing your diabetes?" or "Where does this leave you now?"[2] These are neutral, nonjudgmental questions. It is important for the pharmacist to be very patient during this time of questioning. Patients may vacillate between changing and staying the same.

Principles of Motivational Interviewing

The five principles[5] that are used with the menu of strategies, and a rationale for each principle, are discussed in the following paragraphs.

Express empathy. Practitioners who are judgmental or impatient or perceive the patient as lazy or uncooperative are likely to fail in assisting a patient with change. The pharmacist who sees the patient as one who is struggling with the process of change and respects the patient and the struggle will be far more successful. What you are observing with a patient who seems uncooperative, uninterested, or resistant is that patient's way of coping with the situation. It may not be productive, but it is the only way the patient knows how to cope at the time. One role of the health care provider is to identify and understand the reasons for resistance from the patient's perspective.

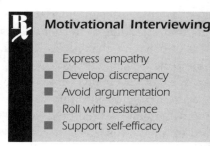

Motivational Interviewing

- Express empathy
- Develop discrepancy
- Avoid argumentation
- Roll with resistance
- Support self-efficacy

Only then can other, more productive ways of coping be identified. The tools successful therapists use to initially assess a patient are open-ended questions, reflective listening, and empathic responding, as described in Chapter 3.

Develop discrepancy. Because patients are often ambivalent about change, initiatives must be taken to begin to move the patient in the direction of the desired change. Although persuasive strategies may work very well for patients in the later stages of change, they fail miserably when patients are in the precontemplation or contemplation stages. Usually, persuasive strategies are met with resistance in these early stages. So, what to do? It has already been suggested that expressing empathy is critical early on. The next step is to develop discrepancies between a patient's present behavior and the behaviors desired. People are much more highly motivated to change when discrepancies exist between current behavior and desired personal goals.[6]

Motivational interviewing attempts to create these discrepancies without making the patient feel threatened or pressured. Through effective questioning, the skilled interviewer attempts to identify existing discrepancies. If this is done properly, the patient will come up with reasons the change is necessary.

Avoid argumentation. As stated by Miller and Rollnick,[5] "Motivational interviewing is confrontational in its purpose: to increase awareness of problems and the need to do something about them." However, this kind of confrontation is different from arguing with the patient, trying to convince patients they have a problem when they are not ready to accept it, or labeling patients (e.g., overweight, diabetic, hypertensive, anorexic, uncooperative) in order to promote change. Arguing tends to increase resistance rather than increasing motivation to change.[1]

Roll with resistance. When dealing with patients who do not want to change, are overwhelmed, or won't take their illnesses seriously, there is a tendency to become frustrated or angry. This frustration or anger often leads to heightened attempts to persuade patients that they have a problem, that they should take it seriously, and that they should make a more committed effort to adhere to the instructions (to "get with the program"). When patients make statements that indicate resistance ("But I just can't remember to take it three times a day," "Yeah, it's easy for you to say. You don't have high blood pressure," "I just don't understand what the big deal is. I feel fine"), they are providing valuable insight into where the problems lie. For example, a less complicated regimen, identification of low-salt foods, or clarification of information may be a solution to the identified problem. Nonetheless, as stated previously, communication that expresses understanding of the problems the patient encounters will go much further than browbeating or arguing. Ultimately, it will be the patient's job (with your support and assistance) to solve the problems presented. You may be able to decrease the complexity of the regimen, but the patient will still have to take the medication. You may be able to suggest foods that are low in sodium, but the patient will still have to avoid high-sodium foods.

Support self-efficacy. Patients have to believe they have the knowledge and skills or abilities to carry out the treatment plan. The pharmacist can help the patient develop self-efficacy about carrying out the treatment plan in various ways:[8] (1) by providing and clarifying information; (2) by offering realistic hope and expressing confidence in the patient's ability to succeed; (3) by noticing successful attempts at adherence, even if they are short-lived; (4) by praising ideas that the patient comes up with to solve problems; and (5) by continuing to emphasize and support the responsibilities that both the patient and the provider have in improving treatment adherence and treatment outcomes.

Dialogue

Let's take a look at a dialogue that shows how we can apply what has been discussed in this chapter. The pharmacist has been trained in motivational interviewing, and the patient, Mrs. Jones, is having a difficult time accepting that she has asthma. Mrs. Jones has brought in several prescriptions.

Mrs. Jones: Here. (quite dejectedly)

Pharmacist: You seem a little down today, Mrs. Jones. (expressing empathy)

Mrs. Jones: Well, look at these prescriptions.

Pharmacist: Looks like you have asthma.

Mrs. Jones: So now you know why I'm so down.

Pharmacist: You are down because you just found out and it came unexpectedly. (expressing empathy)

Mrs. Jones: Well, yes. I mean, I get winded sometimes, but I didn't know I had asthma.

Pharmacist: Asthma sounds bad to you. (expressing empathy)

Mrs. Jones: Sure. You have to take medicine for it. I have to stop smoking. I found out my cat's hair might be a problem. That doesn't sound bad to you?

Pharmacist: It sounds like a lot of change at one time. (expressing empathy and avoiding argumentation)

Mrs. Jones: You're darn right. I might quit smoking, but I've had my little Chubbers for 7 years and I'm not giving her up. I love that cat.

Pharmacist: It sounds like you have a lot of difficult decisions to make. (expressing empathy) What did the doctor tell you about asthma?

Mrs. Jones: Not much. He just said that I need to use these medicines, stop smoking, and get rid of the cat. He's got some nerve—get rid of the cat!

Pharmacist: You didn't like his advice. (expressing empathy, rolling with resistance, and avoiding argumentation)

Mrs. Jones: Not one bit.

Pharmacist: I know that you don't want to get rid of Chubbers. What do you think about quitting smoking?

Mrs. Jones: I don't know. It relaxes me a lot, but Dr. Carroll says it's bad for my asthma. Is that true?

Pharmacist: Smoking does cause asthma to get worse. It does increase your risks associated with asthma.

Mrs. Jones: That's what Dr. Carroll said, too. I guess it's true.

Pharmacist: So, on the one hand you're telling me that smoking relaxes you, but you also seem to be saying that you realize smoking will make your asthma worse. (developing discrepancy)

Mrs. Jones: Yeah, I guess so. I need to go home and sort all of this out. Just fill my prescriptions.

Pharmacist: It all seems somewhat overwhelming right now. (expressing empathy)

Mrs. Jones: Yes.

Pharmacist: I'll get these prescriptions filled and then we'll talk about how to use them properly so you'll get the most benefit from them.

Mrs. Jones: All right.

Pharmacist: Has Dr. Carroll talked to you about a peak flow meter?

Mrs. Jones: A what?

Pharmacist: A peak flow meter to tell how your breathing is doing.

Mrs. Jones: Look, I can't handle anything else right now. Could you just get my prescriptions filled?

Pharmacist: Sure, we can talk about the peak flow meter another time. (rolling with resistance, expressing empathy)

It seems clear from this dialogue that Mrs. Jones is not ready to accept her asthma and the things she may need to do to get it under control. The pharmacist is patient and caring and does not try to push the patient too fast. The pharmacist does not insist on talking to the patient about peak flow because she is not ready to hear about this yet. She is ambivalent about what to do and needs some time to sort things out. The pharmacist uses many of the principles of motivational interviewing in this dialogue. Even though not everything got covered and not every strategy on the menu was used, no bridges were burned and no added resistance occurred, because the pharmacist did not rush things. The pharmacist realized that this is a process and that other opportunities to talk to Mrs. Jones about her asthma would occur.

Summary
Motivational interviewing and the stages of change are useful concepts and processes for meeting patients where they are in their readiness to manage their illnesses. They provide stage-specific skills and strategies for assisting patients with change. They require that pharmacists see their job as serving the needs of the patients, not vice versa. When this can be done, better outcomes are more likely to occur.

Questions for Reflection

1. Why do people have such varied emotional responses to change?
2. Why is ambivalence the biggest cause of resistance to change?
3. Why are persuasive strategies ineffective for people resistant to change?
4. You tell a 50-year-old man with hypertension that he needs to stop smoking. He says, "Look, my grandfather smoked a pack and a half of cigarettes a day and so did my father. They both lived to be 80 years old. Don't worry about it." Using what you have learned in this chapter, discuss what you would say or do in response.
5. How does dissonance increase motivation to change?
6. Describe how patient counseling and motivational interviewing fit together.
7. What are the major components of the transtheoretical model of change? What is the significance of each component?
8. How do motivational interviewing and the transtheoretical model of change fit together?

References

1. Prochaska JO. *Systems of Psychotherapy: A Transtheoretical Approach*. Homewood, Ill: Dorsey Press; 1979.
2. Prochaska JO, DiClemente CC. *The Transtheoretical Approach: Crossing Traditional Boundaries of Therapy*. Homewood, Ill: Dow Jones-Irwin; 1984.
3. DiClemente CC, Prochaska JO, Fairhurst SK, et al. The process of smoking cessation: an analysis of precontemplation, contemplation, and preparation stages of change. *J Consult Clin Psychol*. 1991;59:295–304.
4. DiClemente CC, Prochaska JO, Gibertini M. Self-efficacy and the stages of self-change of smoking. *Cognit Ther Res*. 1985;9:181–200.
5. Miller WR, Rollnick S. *Motivational Interviewing*. New York: Guilford Press; 1991.
6. Rollnick S, Heather N, Bell A. Negotiating behavior change in medical settings: the development of brief motivational interviewing. *J Ment Health*. 1992;1:25–37.
7. Rogers CR. The necessary and sufficient conditions for therapeutic personality change. *J Consult Psychol*. 1957;21:95.
8. Berger BA. *Readiness for Change: Improving Treatment Adherence*. Research Triangle Park, NC: Glaxo Wellcome Inc; 1997.

Chapter 9
INTERACTING WITH PHYSICIANS

With rare exception, the primary reason pharmacists call physicians is that something is wrong or a problem needs to be resolved. Because these calls so often begin with a problem, they can start off in a negative or adversarial way and trigger defensiveness in the physician. But skillful and sensitive pharmacists can turn these negatives into pluses. The provision of pharmaceutical care requires a collaborative relationship with the physician—a relationship in which egos are set aside (you may not be able to control someone else's ego, but you can certainly control your own) and the focus is on preventing and solving drug-related problems with the intent of providing the best possible care for the patient. This means that the focus of any call to the physician (other than those calls that are purely informational) needs to be on assisting the patient and solving or preventing drug-related problems. The relationship must develop out of mutual respect. Calls that are motivated out of a need to "catch someone" or prove a point are not conducive to vital professional relationships. This chapter provides guidelines for discussing drug-related problems with physicians.

Building Rapport

You can build rapport with physicians *before* you need to call them about patients' drug-related problems. Whether you are an independent pharmacy owner or an employee pharmacist, it is important to rethink who you are and what you do. Are you a health care provider? Do you have a practice? Or do you simply see yourself as someone who fills prescriptions? If you do see yourself as a health care provider with a practice, then meeting with local physicians is a vital step in building rapport and allowing you to be more effective in drug therapy decision-making. As suggested in the book *A Practical Guide to Pharmaceutical Care*,[1] pharmacists can meet with local physicians to

- Inform them of new service offerings and your desire to work together to benefit patients. It is important to explain the benefit of each new service to physicians in a way that emphasizes what is in it for them. For example, let's say that you are going to develop educational services and sessions for asthma patients. Point out to the physician (particularly general practitioners and family practitioners) that you understand how busy they are and know that often they do not have time to be as thorough as they would like. By providing this service and working collaboratively with the physician, you can keep the patient's asthma under control so that the patient does not need to switch to a specialist (pulmonologist). One pharmacist sold the idea for a blood pressure monitoring service to a physician on the basis that every 2 weeks he would fax or e-mail the patient's readings to the physician, along with brief notes. This way the physician, who saw the patient only every 3 to 6 months, would have better information at his disposal.

- Encourage physicians to discuss what services would assist them in their practice.
- Discuss changes that are taking place in pharmacy in general that could lead to better care for patients.
- Update them on new drug developments within a specialty area or in general. Providing physicians with unbiased information about new products can be very useful from both an efficacy and a cost perspective. It can also elevate your status as a pharmacist and that of the profession.

Pharmacists who cannot meet face-to-face with local physicians can send a letter introducing themselves and their new services. The letter can ask physicians to indicate what services they desire and whether they would be willing to meet and discuss these services further. Whether the contact is face-to-face or through a letter, it helps build rapport and credibility and separates you from everyone else.

Reasons for Calling

Pharmacists usually contact physicians about the following types of drug-related problems:

> The focus of any call to the physician...needs to be on assisting the patient and solving or preventing drug-related problems.

- Untreated condition(s). The patient needs drug therapy but is not receiving it.
- Improper drug selection. In addition to a wrong drug for this patient and indication, improper selection could mean that the patient can't afford the drug or is allergic to the drug, that the drug hasn't helped or been tolerated in the past, or that the patient has renal or hepatic impairment that makes the drug choice improper.
- Dosage too high. The wrong dose, frequency, or duration or a drug interaction could make the dose too high.
- Subtherapeutic dosage. This could result from a wrong dose, frequency, or duration; a drug interaction; or storage or administration that lowers the effective dose.
- Adverse drug reactions and side effects that cannot be tolerated or won't go away. This could result from inappropriate dosing or administration or from drug interactions.
- Drug interactions.
- Unnecessary drug therapy. This could include drug use without a medical indication, addiction or recreational drug use, situations in which nondrug

therapy or no therapy is more appropriate, duplicate therapy, or treating an avoidable adverse reaction to another drug.

- Compliance problems. These can occur when the patient cannot tolerate side effects, the cost is too high, the dosage regimen is too frequent or complex, the patient cannot swallow or otherwise administer the drug, the patient does not understand how the drug works or how to take it, or the patient does not understand the need for the drug or the severity of the illness.

Other reasons for contacting the physician include

- Inability to read or interpret a prescription order,
- Request to change a drug and suggestion for a therapeutic alternative because a product is out of stock, a specific brand is necessary, or the patient can't afford, is allergic to, or has not been helped in the past by the prescribed drug,
- Refill authorization,
- Request for additional information about the patient for your database, and
- Physician detailing or counterdetailing to introduce important new products or new services in your pharmacy.

Preparation before Calling

Pharmacist–physician communication can be frustrating for both parties when the pharmacist has not prepared adequately. Before contacting the physician, you need to consider the following points:

- Have the necessary facts ready, including your recommendation and rationale. These facts include not only drug- and disease-related information but relevant patient information (e.g., the patient cannot afford the drug, can't remember to take it, cannot tolerate side effects).
- Have a literature citation ready, if possible (use the Web or hard-copy references).
- Know what you're talking about. Don't waste a busy physician's time. Be succinct and to the point in your communication. Identify yourself (Hi, this is Tina King at The Apothecary), the patient involved (Ruth Jones), the problem (is still getting heartburn and it's keeping her up at night), and your recommendation (therefore, I would like to recommend that we switch her from X to Y). Provide any other relevant information (she has taken her X as prescribed and cut down on fatty and spicy food, and she does not eat close to bedtime, yet she is not getting much relief).
- Get sufficient information from the patient (what the problem is as the patient sees it) to be prepared.
- Be prepared to use the SOAP approach (subjective and objective information, assessment, and plan), because this is what physicians are accustomed to.

■ Always have an alternative recommendation ready in case your initial recommendation is not accepted.

Communication Considerations

Before contacting the physician, consider the following communication strategies.

The entire focus should be on attacking problems or issues, not people or personalities. Keep the focus of the conversation on solving patient problems, not on pointing out that the drug therapy prescribed is inappropriate. There is a big difference between the following statements: "Dr. Smith, Mrs. Jones can't use those tablets you prescribed" and "Dr. Smith, Mrs. Jones has trouble swallowing. I would like to recommend..." The latter is far more likely to elicit cooperation, because it states the problem in terms of Mrs. Jones's swallowing difficulties, not what Dr. Smith did. For another example, rather than saying, "You shouldn't have prescribed X because Mrs. Jones is taking Y and the two drugs interact," say, "Because Mrs. Jones is already taking Y, I'm concerned about her getting X because of the drug interaction. I suggest we use Z instead for the following reasons..."

Make sure professional boundaries are respected; this goes both ways. Don't try to play doctor, and don't second-guess the doctor. Ask questions and show interest in the patient, not in being right.

Mentally and emotionally prepare for different consequences. What will you say if you are met with resistance, anger, belligerence, attempts at intimidation, or refusal? To what extent are you willing to persist and not back down?

Use a combination of information exchange, assertiveness, and effective listening. Make sure that you listen completely to the physician's rationale for the decisions made. Repeat back your understanding, and be prepared to offer an alternative in a confident, assertive, nonjudgmental manner.

For telephone communication, be prepared to talk to a nurse or member of the office staff. You may need to assert yourself if you need to speak to the physician. Think about what conditions would necessitate talking directly to the physician.

Use 4F communication: "I know how you *feel*. I *felt* the same way, too. But I *found* in the literature...," and stay *focused* on the problem.

Table 9-1 provides guidelines for contacting physicians in person and by telephone. Two sample dialogues about the same drug therapy problem are given at the end of the chapter.

Table 9-1. Guidelines for Contacting Physicians

	In Person	By Telephone
State who you are and the purpose of the call (be pleasant)	"Hi, Dr. Jones. I'm Joe Smith, one of the pharmacists here. I need to talk to you about Carla Brown's prescription for (name of medication). Is this a good time?" When the call is urgent, don't ask if it's a good time.	"Hi, I'm Joe Smith from Smith's Pharmacy. I need to talk to Dr. Jones about Carla Brown's prescription."
State the problem and recom-mended solution	"You prescribed (name of medication) for Carla. She does not have any third-party coverage and would have to pay for this medication out of her own pocket. She says she cannot afford it. I would like to recommend (name of medication) if you are treating (indication). This would be affordable to her and would be equally or nearly as effective." If you are not sure what is being treated, ask for the indication and be prepared to make a recom-mendation.	"Dr. Jones wrote a prescription for Carla for (name of medication). She does not have any third-party coverage and would have to pay for this medication out of her own pocket. She says she cannot afford it. I would like to recom-mend (name of medication) if Dr. Jones is treating (indication). This would be affordable to her and would be equally or nearly as effective." If you are not sure what is being treated, ask for the indication and be prepared to make a recommendation.
If you meet resistance	Stay focused on the problem. Make good eye contact. Repeat back your understanding of what the physician's resistance is about. "So, if I understand you correctly, you simply don't like using (name of medication you recommended) because you have had better success with (name of medication)." The physician confirms this, and you state, "Given that you are treating (indication), I have found (give citation) that (name of medication recommended) is very effective. I'm very concerned that Ms. Brown won't take the (name of medication) because it is too expensive for her. I have tried to convince her that it might prevent future visits, but she insists she won't take it. Can we try the (name of medication recommended)?"	Stay focused on the problem. Repeat back your understanding of what the physician's resistance is about. "So, if I understand you correctly, you simply don't like using (name of medication you recommended) because you have had better success with (name of medication)." The physician confirms this, and you state, "Given that you are treating (indication), I have found (give citation) that (name of medication recommended) is very effective. I'm very concerned that Ms. Brown won't take the (name of medication) because it is too expensive for her. I have tried to convince her that it might prevent future visits, but she insists she won't take it. Can we try the (name of medication recommended)?"

Contingencies

When a physician refuses to take your recommendation to change an order, don't continue to argue. Simply tell the patient what happened. Identify alternatives, if possible. When a patient may be harmed by inappropriate therapy and the physician refuses to change the order, state, "Dr. Jones, I cannot in good conscience give Ms. Brown this medication, because I believe it is harmful to her. I will not dispense it. Again, I recommend (name of medication). If this is not acceptable, I will simply explain to her why I cannot dispense the (name of medication)." Don't attempt, in any way, to make the physician look bad to the patient, even if you are correct about your recommendation. You can only lose in such an interchange. Stick with the facts, what you told the physician, what you recommended, and what you think should be done now.

Involving the Patient

In general, whenever a physician needs to be contacted about a problem with a patient's drug therapy, the patient should be involved. However, we have to be careful not to jeopardize the physician–patient relationship. For example, a patient is prescribed an appetite suppressant by a physician who does not know the patient has high blood pressure. It is important to inform the patient that you need to call the physician treating her high blood pressure to discuss this new medication, and the reason for the call. Emphasize that you understand that the prescriber did not realize she has high blood pressure. Consider what you would do if the patient asked you not to call her physician because she didn't want to bother him and told you that she would talk to her doctor. If she insisted on this, it would be important to not dispense any medication that could harm her and to put in writing what the problem is and what solution you propose. Make a copy for the patient and keep a copy in your files. In this way, your communication to the patient won't be communicated to the physician incorrectly or incompletely.

Pulling Things Together

Now let's take a look at two pharmacist–physician dialogues about the same problem. These dialogues indicate how preparation, focus, and interpersonal skills can make a great deal of difference.

Dialogue 1

Pharmacist: Yeah, doc, the amoxicillin you prescribed for Mrs. Tanner's kid is not working. We need to get her something else.

Physician: Who is this?

Pharmacist: Joe at Conners Drugs—the pharmacist.

Physician: What do you mean it's not working? Did she give it to the child correctly? He's only been taking it for 5 or 6 days. She has a 10-day supply. Is the child still running a fever?

Pharmacist: I guess she's giving it to him right. She says he's not feeling good and she wants to give him something else. I didn't ask about a fever.

Physician: Tell her to call me. I'll take care of it.

Pharmacist: You got it, doc!

Discussion

This pharmacist was not prepared. He simply didn't do his homework before he called. In addition, he defined the problem as the drug prescribed by the physician. The problem is that the patient was not getting better (as defined by the mother). The pharmacist did not have clear information to support the contention that there was a problem. As a result, the physician decided to talk to the patient directly rather than waste any more time talking to an ill-prepared pharmacist. This conversation reflects poorly on the individual pharmacist and the profession.

Let's look at how this might have been approached.

Dialogue 2

Pharmacist: Hi, Dr. Smith. This is Sara Thomas, a pharmacist at Conners Drugs. I just got off the phone with Susan Tanner, Brady's mother. She called because she was concerned about Brady. His fever is still at 101.5 and he has been taking the amoxicillin for 6 days now, three times a day as you prescribed. She said he's pretty miserable. I assumed that Brady has otitis because she talked about his ear infection and I saw from his medication record that he was treated for otitis once before, about 3 months ago. I think it might be time to go to trimethoprim–sulfamethoxazole twice a day or cefaclor every 8 to 12 hours.

Physician: So he's still running a fever. From what you have said it sounds like he's not responding to the amoxicillin. OK, give him the trimethoprim–sulfamethoxazole twice a day. Do you have his weight?

Pharmacist: Sure do.

Physician: Good. Let's keep him on it for 10 days.

Pharmacist: OK. I'll let Mrs. Tanner know.

Physician: Thanks for calling.

Pharmacist: You're welcome. Thanks for getting back to me so quickly.

Discussion

This pharmacist was well prepared and kept her focus on the problem. She gave the physician more than one option and, as a result of her thoroughness, the physician was able to make a decision quickly. Although all situations may not go as smoothly, they are far more likely to go this way with preparation and appropriate focus.

Summary

It is often uncomfortable for pharmacists to call physicians, since the nature of the call is that there is a problem. Well-prepared, skilled pharmacists who focus on patient problems rather than on prescribing problems can turn these calls into opportunities for professional collaboration and cooperation, rather than conflict.

Questions for Reflection

1. When calling a physician about a potential drug-related problem, what preparation do you need before making the call?
2. Rephrase the following statement: "Dr. Smith, the medicine you prescribed for Mrs. Jones's arthritis is not doing a thing for her. What do you want to do?"
3. What should you do if a physician refuses to make a drug therapy change and you know that the prescribed drug is inappropriate for the patient? Describe what you would say and what steps you would take.
4. It has been said that pharmaceutical care cannot be accomplished without pharmacists establishing collaborative relationships with physicians. What would this involve?
5. In what ways can you get local physicians more involved in changes that you want to accomplish in your practice?

Reference

1. Rovers JP, Currie JD, Hagel HP, et al. *A Practical Guide to Pharmaceutical Care.* Washington, DC: American Pharmaceutical Association; 1998:91.

Chapter 10
SUPPORTIVE COMMUNICATION

It is fairly common for patients to come to the pharmacy and present a prescription and then say or do something that indicates they are distressed. The distress is often related to whatever problem the prescription is attempting to solve or alleviate. Sometimes the distress is related to some other event or events. Because the pharmacist is a health care provider—one who is supposed to render care—it seems reasonable to expect pharmacists to be able to respond in these situations in a way that communicates caring, concern, or comfort to the patient. This is supportive communication.

In this chapter, we will examine the benefits of supportive communication, different ways to respond with supportive communication, problems associated with supportive communication, and unsupportive or unhelpful messages. Many of the ideas and concepts in this chapter are derived from the work of Albrecht, Burleson, and Goldsmith.[1] Readers can find more information on the subject in that outstanding reference.

Need for Supportive Communication

As stated by Basch,[2] "though we tend not to be aware of it, the need to communicate on some level with other human beings—that is, to make ourselves understood or understandable, and in doing so feel cared for, safe, stimulated, and appreciated—remains the prime motivator for all that we do or don't do." Supportive communication allows people to feel understood and less alone.

Squier[3] discussed the importance of practitioner understanding in predicting treatment adherence. According to Squier, (1) patient adherence was higher when physicians allowed patients to express and dissipate their tensions and anxiety about their illness and when physicians took the time to carefully answer the patient's questions; (2) practitioners who demonstrated responsiveness to patients' feelings had patients with higher adherence rates and better satisfaction with the relationship; (3) patients who perceived their physicians as understanding and caring were more likely to carry out the treatment plan and ask for further help or advice when they needed it; and (4) health care providers who encouraged patients' expressions of feelings and participation in the treatment plan were found to have patients with higher rates of adherence. These are important findings with significant implications for pharmacy practice. Again, feeling understood strengthens the relationship between the patient and the provider. This may improve treatment adherence and encourage the patient to continue to frequent the pharmacy. In addition to the emotional and psychological benefits, supportive communication has been demonstrated to have physical and health benefits, improve resistance to infection and disease, and extend life.[1]

Types of Supportive Communication

This discussion will focus on responding supportively when patients are distressed. This type of interaction is often difficult for people, because they want to be supportive and sometimes aren't sure what to say or how to say it. Although it is equally important to respond to people when they are expressing happiness or joy, most of us are fairly comfortable about responding to people when they are in a good mood. In either case, the key is to understand the validity and importance of the feelings being expressed.

Patients often express sadness when they find out they have a chronic illness, like diabetes, high blood pressure, or asthma. Their sadness results from a feeling of loss. The loss, usually permanent, involves losing something good, desirable, or pleasurable from the patient's perspective. The loss could involve needing to give up certain foods. It could mean needing to give up certain habits, such as smoking. Although most health care providers would agree that smoking is not a good thing, it still may be pleasurable or relaxing to the patient. The loss might also involve a general sense of loss of invincibility. A chronic illness reminds us that we are growing old and won't live forever.

When a patient is saddened by such losses, the purpose of supportive communication is to help the patient accept the loss. This is done by legitimizing the patient's feelings, acknowledging the importance and permanence of the loss to the patient, and encouraging the patient to accept the loss.[3] Let's look at an example:

Patient: I thought I just had some allergies. Now I find out I have asthma. Doc says I have to give up smoking. It's one of the few things that relaxes me.

Pharmacist: It sounds like finding out about asthma has been difficult for you. It could be very hard to stop smoking, since it's so relaxing for you. That would certainly help your asthma, though.

Patient: Yeah, I know. It's just tough.

Pharmacist: It sounds difficult.

> **Your job is to demonstrate caring and concern for the patient—not to solve the patient's problems.**

Note that this pharmacist does not try to make everything better. The pharmacist doesn't try to cheer up the patient and point out all the benefits of not smoking and all the good things in the patient's life. It's too soon for that. That may be useful at some point, but not now.

Becoming ill also evokes fear and anxiety in patients. These two emotions occur because the patient experiences ambivalence, circumstances seem uncontrollable, or there is a perceived or real threat to the patient. The same illness that produces sadness in one patient may produce fear or anxiety in another patient. Therefore, pharmacists must be sensitive to how each patient uniquely processes the illness and its treatment. For patients who are fearful or anxious, supportive communication focuses on legitimizing the feelings of the patient, "reducing the individual's uncertainty about the situation, enhancing the individual's sense of efficacy or control, modifying judgments about the harmfulness of a perceived threat, or identifying ways to escape from the threat."[1] Here's an example:

Patient: The doctor told me I have high blood pressure. Am I gonna have a heart attack?

Pharmacist: This must be very frightening for you. It's true that patients who have uncontrolled high blood pressure for a sustained period of time are at a higher risk for a heart attack, but the medicine your doctor has prescribed is very effective at controlling blood pressure if it's taken once a day as prescribed.

Patient: So, if I take this, I won't have a heart attack?

Pharmacist: I feel very confident that if you take this medicine properly, cut down on salt in your diet, and get some moderate exercise on a regular basis you will greatly reduce the risk of a heart attack. It really is up to you. I know these are things that you can handle without a problem.

Patient: I hope so.

The pharmacist in this situation legitimized the patient's concern, then gave the patient a realistic appraisal of the risks of a heart attack. The pharmacist helped to reduce uncertainty by letting the patient know about those things that are under his control, then supported the self-efficacy of the patient by letting him know that he could do what is necessary to escape the threat of a heart attack.

Shame, embarrassment, and guilt are other emotions that are evoked by one's own illness and the illness of loved ones. Shame and embarrassment result from feeling "caught" when you don't want to be caught. Shame or embarrassment occurs when a person's character or competence is questioned (either privately or publicly)—when the person's self-image is either challenged or confirmed (some people already believe they are not competent or worthy of respect). If a patient is treated like a child and shamed by a physician for not following her treatment plan correctly (in the eyes of the physician), that shame may have been converted to anger or intolerance by the time she reaches the pharmacy. This is a very difficult situation. Supportive communication is needed to let the patient know that she still deserves to be treated with respect, regardless of whether she followed the treatment regimen. But the patient's anger or intolerance may be met with far less than supportive communication by the pharmacist. The key for the pharmacist is to stay separate from the patient—that is, to not be taken in by the patient's anger. Here is an example:

Patient: Here, fill this! (tosses prescription on the counter angrily)

Pharmacist: Sounds like this has been a difficult day.

Patient: Hmmf. Difficult day...you people think it's so easy to take all of this medicine and change your whole life when you get ill!

Pharmacist: I hope I haven't given you that impression. I know that keeping your diabetes under control takes a lot of effort and hard work.

Patient: You're darn right it does. Tell that to Dr. Harris.

Pharmacist: You don't think he understands that?

Patient: Not a bit. I don't deserve to be belittled like a child because my weight isn't where he thinks it ought to be.

Pharmacist: Sounds like you had a very difficult time with Dr. Harris today.

Patient: He has no idea how hard I've tried.

Pharmacist: You really have tried hard.

Patient: Yes, I have.

In this situation, the pharmacist does not take the patient's anger personally. He supports the patient without taking sides and without assuming that the patient's story about Dr. Harris is accurate or inaccurate. The pharmacist simply responds to what the patient is having difficulty with and supports her character.

Guilt arises when people believe they did something they should not have done or didn't do something they should have done. A feeling of helplessness goes with guilt. The goal of supportive communication in dealing with another's guilt feelings is to first acknowledge the feeling and then ask what the other person thinks he or she can do to change those feelings of guilt. Finally, support and encourage the action steps the person identifies.

Patient's mother: I just wish I would have checked his peak flow more often. If I had, he wouldn't have had to go to the emergency room again. I could have done something. He's only 9 years old, and he's been through so much.

Pharmacist: You're feeling somewhat responsible for his needing to go to the emergency room.

Patient's mother: Well, sure. I'm his mother.

Pharmacist: It's hard to see these things happen to your child. What do you think you can do to prevent this from happening?

Patient's mother: I need to chart his peak flow, like you said, and use his medicines accordingly. I need to stick with this.

Pharmacist: I think those are very good ideas. It might also help to involve him in charting the peak flow readings and have him remind you if you forget. He's old enough to be taking some responsibility.

Patient's mother: OK. That's a good idea.

The pharmacist acknowledges the mother's feelings and does not attempt to smooth things over and make everything all right. He allows the patient's mother to come up with solutions and supports them. Finally, he also interjects that some of the responsibility could be shared by the child.

Anger is another emotion that is difficult for most people to confront. We simply want it to stop, and our communication often conveys that. (For a more complete discussion of managing anger, see Chapter 5.) This can backfire. Anger is a response to a blocked goal or some sense of injustice. As with shame and embarrassment, anger is often a substitute for some other feeling (e.g., fear, frustration, hurt), because anger feels more powerful and less helpless or weak than those other feelings. Supportive communication attempts to acknowledge the legitimacy of the other person's feelings, help identify ways to reach blocked goals, and support the other person when it seems clear that an injustice has been done.

Patient: Fifteen minutes just to throw a few pills in a bottle! I don't have all day. All I do is wait on you people! First at the doctor's office, now here, and I'm late for an appointment.

Pharmacist: I know that all of this can be very frustrating. Would you like to use the phone to let them know you're running late for your next appointment, or perhaps pick up your prescription later?

Patient: I'm just tired of waiting. I waited almost an hour past my appointment time in the doctor's office.

Pharmacist: I don't like that either. We're all busy, not just the doctor. I will do my best to get this prescription ready as quickly as I can.

Patient: Just hurry.

The pharmacist acknowledges the patient's feelings but does not take the patient's anger personally. The pharmacist offers the patient some options (for reaching a blocked goal) and reassures the patient that she will get the prescription filled as quickly as possible. In addition, the pharmacist offers support (for an injustice) by letting the patient know that she too dislikes it when physicians (and others) don't stay on time for their appointments.

Table 10-1 summarizes this discussion on emotions and supportive communication. Regardless of the feeling expressed, supportive communication attempts to legitimize the other's feelings.

Problems Associated with Supportive Communication

There are three major problems associated with supportive communication: (1) no matter what you do or say, the other person can decide to remain angry, indifferent, or uncooperative; (2) defenses resulting from certain situations or conditions can cause patients to displace a core emotion and replace it with anger or indifference at a time when they most need support; and (3) supportive communication takes time, effort, and practice.

First, it needs to be clear that your job is to demonstrate caring and concern for the patient—*not* to solve the patient's problems, especially if the problems were created long before your relationship with the patient began. For example, if a patient is running late for an appointment, the pharmacist can help as much as possible by providing care to the patient quickly. However, the pharmacist did not make the patient late and should not accept being chastised by the patient because the patient

Table 10-1. Emotions and Supportive Communication

Emotion	Resulting from	Supportive Communication Goals
Sadness	Sense of permanent loss	1. Legitimize the feelings of the other. 2. Acknowledge the importance and permanence of the loss. 3. Encourage the patient to accept the loss.
Fear, anxiety	Ambivalence, circumstances that seem uncontrollable, a perceived or real threat	1. Legitimize the feelings of the other. 2. Reduce the individual's uncertainty about the situation. 3. Enhance the individual's sense of control or efficacy. 4. Modify judgments about the harmfulness of a perceived threat. 5. Identify ways to escape from the threat.
Shame or embarrassment	Feeling caught, having one's character or competence questioned	1. Legitimize the feelings of the other. 2. Support the character or competence of the other.
Guilt	Doing something that should not have been done or not doing something that should have been done	1. Acknowledge the feeling. 2. Ask what the other thinks he or she can do to change the feelings of guilt. 3. Support and encourage action steps identified by the other.
Anger	Blocked goals, sense of injustice	1. Acknowledge the legitimacy of the other's feelings. 2. Help identify ways to reach blocked goals. 3. Support the other when it seems clear that an injustice has been done.

is late. Some people, at some times, will not respond to caring and concern no matter how it is demonstrated. At such times it becomes necessary to either move on or, for example, to assertively ask the patient to stop yelling at you. You cannot be made responsible for others' incivility, regardless of the reason.

Second, certain illnesses (like depression), some emotions (like shame), and certain conditions (like stigmatization of HIV or AIDS) cause patients to feel so uncomfortable and hurt that they convert this hurt to feeling angry or more withdrawn. They are in great need of social support and supportive communication, yet their own anger, discomfort, or withdrawal evokes discomfort in others (including health care providers) to the point where they respond with anger or avoidance when the patient most needs support and confirmation. Our angry response or withdrawal can exacerbate the patient's feelings of isolation. There is no simple solution here.

Start by keeping in mind, regardless of the emotional display of the patient, that we can focus on legitimizing feelings and listening carefully without feeling responsible for the patient's feelings or condition. This is difficult, but essential.

> **Supportive communication allows people to feel understood and less alone.**

Third, the skills we have been discussing require that a certain amount of uninterrupted time be spent with the patient. In some community pharmacy settings, this is difficult. But not using these skills leads to even greater expenditures of time. It takes practice and sensitivity in listening to the patient for these skills to be mastered and used effectively, so patience with yourself is also required.

Unhelpful or Unsupportive Messages

When interacting with patients who are distressed, health care providers can engage in unhelpful or unsupportive communication by being indifferent or overly concerned or helpful, by not listening carefully, or by trying to fix the problem or the patient. If we intend to truly provide care, indifference is unacceptable when interacting with a distressed patient.

Being overly concerned can be suffocating to the patient or can exacerbate the patient's belief about being weak by admitting to a problem in the first place. When we are overly concerned, it is usually because we are trying to take care of our own needs (the need to be seen as helpful, nice, or good) rather than focusing on what the patient needs. Some patients simply may not be ready for any assistance.

When we try to fix the problem or the patient, it is usually because we are uncomfortable with the patient or problem and want the patient or the problem to go away as soon as possible. Learning to simply listen and legitimize feelings rather than trying to solve a problem or cheer a patient up will alleviate some of the stress associated with hearing about people's problems.

Summary

Supportive communication is an essential part of building a trusting therapeutic relationship with the patient. For supportive communication to be effective, the pharmacist must listen to the feeling expressed by the patient, be aware of what that feeling results from, and use supportive messages that address the issues that elicited the specific feeling (see Table 10-1). This will result in more satisfying and longer-lasting relationships with patients.

Questions for Reflection

1. Explain why it is that sometimes when people are in most need of supportive communication, their behavior pushes others away.
2. Why do different emotions require different supportive responses?
3. Why do health care providers often have problems with supportive communication?
4. Distinguish the types of responses needed by a patient who is hurt and one who is sad.
5. What should you do if your attempts at supportive communication are met with hostility or indifference by a patient?

References

1. Albrecht TL, Burleson BR, Goldsmith D. Supportive communication. In: Knapp ML, Miller GR, eds. *Handbook of Interpersonal Communication.* 2nd ed. Thousand Oaks, Calif: Sage Publications; 1994.
2. Basch MF. Empathic understanding: a review of the concept and some theoretical considerations. *J Am Psychoanal Assoc.* 1983;31:101–26.
3. Squier RW. A model of empathic understanding and adherence to treatment regimens in practitioner–patient relationships. *Soc Sci Med.* 1990;30:325–39.

Chapter 11
CHOOSING AN APPROPRIATE RESPONSE

This chapter summarizes different types of responses to patients and the benefits and downsides of each type. The purpose is to help you choose a response that is the most appropriate for a particular situation in your practice. Table 11-1 lists each type of response and gives an example of each, along with the benefits and downside of the response.

Our responses to our patients should be motivated by a willingness to help or care for the patient, not a need to reduce our own anxiety, fear, or frustration because of what a patient says or does. If we are uncomfortable at times, this should be instructive to us, not a stimulus to do whatever we can to escape our discomfort. Our frame of reference should be one of serving the client's needs, not our own. From this perspective we can best assess whether our responses are appropriate or inappropriate. Our major focus is helping patients to[1]

1. Feel understood and accepted, thereby allowing them to more freely and openly discuss their problems,
2. Achieve an increased and more accurate understanding of their situation,
3. Discuss alternatives, where necessary,
4. Make decisions about next steps, along with specific actions to be taken, and
5. Make adjustments so that the best results can be obtained.

Table 11-1. Types of Responses and Their Benefits and Downsides

Response and Example	Benefits	Downsides
Empathy: An objective identification with the affective state of an individual **Patient:** (looking very concerned) "Even though the doctor says the stress test is just routine, I know I am very ill. The nurse read my chart and had a very alarmed look on her face. I know something is terribly wrong."	Most helpful in developing a therapeutic relationship. Allows the patient to feel understood, less alone or "crazy."	Sometimes can be painful, yet the suffering is generally useful to the patient.

continued on page 120

Table 11-1. Types of Responses, continued

Response and Example	Benefits	Downsides
Pharmacist: "You're worried that something is seriously wrong and the doctor and nurse aren't telling you everything."		
Reassurance: An attempt to make the patient feel better or more confident **Patient:** "I can't believe that I have high blood pressure." **Pharmacist:** "Don't worry, it'll be OK."	May be exactly what the patient wants to hear, but use only when the patient asks for it ("Do others feel this way?").	Runs the risk of ignoring or minimizing the patient's feelings. You never find out how the patient uniquely sees the problem.
Probing or questioning: An attempt to obtain additional information **Patient:** "The doctor was so rude. I'm not crazy. My neck really does hurt." **Pharmacist:** "Have you thought about seeing another doctor?" or "How long has your neck been hurting?"	Useful when additional information is needed in order to draw appropriate conclusions.	The patient's feelings are ignored. Not very useful where content involves expression of feelings.
Advising: Providing information to assist in solving a problem—depends on who is the expert **Patient:** "What do you recommend for small cuts?" **Pharmacist:** "I recommend this antibiotic ointment."	When the pharmacist is the expert on solving the problem, this is very useful.	Not particularly useful when the patient is the expert ("Should I let my mother-in-law come stay with us over the holidays?").
Generalizing or comparing: An attempt to state what is generally true **Patient:** "I can't believe I have high blood pressure." **Pharmacist:** "Millions of people have high blood pressure and do just fine."	May be exactly what the patient wants to hear.	Runs the risk of ignoring or minimizing the patient's feelings. You never find out how the patient uniquely sees the problem.

continued on page 121

Table 11-1. Types of Responses, continued

Response and Example	Benefits	Downsides
Assertiveness: A response in which the patient and the pharmacist are respected **Patient:** "This is idiotic. Fifteen minutes is ridiculous. I shouldn't have to wait this long to get a prescription filled!" **Pharmacist:** "Fifteen minutes can be a long time when you are in a hurry. However, I do have three other patients ahead of you, and I want to be as thorough and as accurate as possible. So, it will take 15 minutes."	Keeps the subjective, judgmental aspects out of the communication. Allows for deflection of criticism without loss of self-respect or respect for the patient. Allows for differing viewpoints to be acknowledged.	When people want to be "crazy," it can sometimes make them act crazier because they do not want to accept a reasonable response.
Aggressiveness: A response that does not respect the other's viewpoints or actions **Patient:** "This is idiotic. Fifteen minutes is ridiculous. I shouldn't have to wait this long to get a prescription filled!" **Pharmacist:** "This isn't fast food here. What we do is important, and I don't need you yelling at me!"	None—temporary feeling of victory.	May cause problem or anger to escalate.
Nonassertiveness: A response in which you fail to respect yourself **Patient:** "This is idiotic. Fifteen minutes is ridiculous. I shouldn't have to wait this long to get a prescription filled!" **Pharmacist:** "You're right. You shouldn't have to wait so long. I'll get your prescription right away."	The patient may get what he or she wants.	You feel like you have a "kick me" sign on your back. The patient may attempt to take advantage of you in the future.

continued on page 122

Table 11-1. Types of Responses, continued

Response and Example	Benefits	Downsides
Judging: Any message that indicates to the patient that he or she is wrong or shouldn't act or feel as he or she does **Patient:** "The doctor makes me wait all that time and then hurries me through once I finally get to see him." **Pharmacist:** "You have to understand how busy the doctor is."	None.	Does not acknowledge the patient's feelings. May be demeaning.

Empathy

An empathic response is used to convey caring and an accurate understanding of the affective state of another. It is offered objectively, so that the person's feelings are accurately reflected back without any judgment about the appropriateness of those feelings. The feelings are simply a reflection of how the other is responding affectively to a situation, which is not good or bad. An empathic response allows people to feel understood and safe in talking about a concern or even something they like or enjoy. The only possible downside to empathy is that your characterization of the person's feelings can prompt the person to "let go" and feel even more intensely. This can be painful or sometimes frightening, even though it is therapeutic and helps the person move forward. Here are two examples:

EXAMPLE 1

Patient: You and my doctor are only interested in getting my money.

Pharmacist: You are angry because it seems like your doctor and I care more about your money than about you.

EXAMPLE 2

Patient: I just found out I have diabetes. I knew something was wrong.

Pharmacist: You knew something was wrong, but you weren't prepared to find out you have diabetes. This worries you.

Reassurance

A reassuring response attempts to make someone feel better, relieved, less frightened, or more confident. Although such responses are attempts to help or care, they are often motivated by the anxiety of the person providing them. That is, one person says something that indicates he or she feels frightened or overwhelmed. The other person gives a reassuring response ("Don't worry, it'll be OK") in an attempt to relieve his or her own anxiety about not knowing how to help or alleviate the problem. Reassuring responses work best when the other person asks for reassurance. They can backfire when the person does not ask for reassurance and really just wants to be understood. The following two examples should clarify this.

EXAMPLE 1

Patient: Have other patients told you they were afraid to give themselves allergy shots?

Pharmacist: They sure have. I feel confident that, like other patients, you'll have no problem with it after some practice. I'll be glad to show you how to do it.

Patient: Great. I'd like that. Thanks.

Reassurance worked here because the patient asked for it. The patient did not want to feel alone in her fear, so she asked if other patients had this problem. She needed reassurance that she was not alone in being afraid.

EXAMPLE 2

Patient: I just feel so overwhelmed. I finally get my blood pressure under control and now I find out I have asthma. What next?

Pharmacist: Mrs. Smith, it's not so bad. Asthma can be controlled. You'll be OK.

Patient: What do you mean, it's not so bad? Do you have high blood pressure? Do you have asthma? It's easy for you to stand there and say it's not so bad!

Pharmacist: Calm down. It's going to be all right.

Patient: Don't tell me to calm down! This isn't happening to you.

What happened here? Was the pharmacist trying to be caring? The pharmacist wanted to show caring, but his responses were motivated by his anxiety and his desire to fix the problem rather than simply be emotionally available to Mrs. Smith. The pharmacist hoped that if he could fix the problem, he would not have to feel anxious. Mrs. Smith's reaction shows that this did not happen.

Probing or Questioning

This type of response, particularly if questions are open-ended, is useful when you are interested in receiving information from the patient or from the patient's perspective. This type of response usually works well when factual information is needed, but it can be problematic when emotional issues are involved.

EXAMPLE 1

Patient's mother: I don't know what to do. She's been coughing like this for a while.

Pharmacist: I know you're worried about Sara. When did you first notice the cough?

Patient's mother: About 3 days ago.

Pharmacist: Please tell me about any other symptoms you've noticed, like fever or sore throat.

As you can see, probing and questioning here are very important for gathering information so that an informed decision can be made about a product recommendation or referral to a physician. Notice that the pharmacist first acknowledged the mother's concern. Let's look at a situation where this type of response may not be very effective.

EXAMPLE 2

Patient: Thirty-five dollars? You're kidding. I can't afford that!

Pharmacist: Don't you think you're worth it?

Patient: That's not the point. It's a lot of money.

Pharmacist: And don't you think that helping your arthritis is worth $35? I'm sure you've spent more money on less important things than your health.

Patient: I can't believe this. Where do you get off?

Obviously, probing and questioning did not work here. That's because there was no attempt to understand the patient's perspective. In fact, the questioning was manipulative and was really an attempt to bully the patient, even though it was disguised as being reasonable. Too often, we use probing and questioning to "get the facts," when seeking first to understand the world from the patient's perspective would be more beneficial.

Advising

As with many of the other responses, there are times when advising is appropriate and times when it is not. In general, advising is appropriate when you are clearly the expert. Otherwise, advising should be avoided or used very cautiously. Let's look at two examples.

EXAMPLE 1

Patient: I have some burning and itching between my toes. Do you think it could be athlete's foot? (Patient is wearing sandals and pharmacist examines his feet.)

Pharmacist: It sure looks like it. I highly recommend this product (hands it to patient). It is very effective against athlete's foot fungus. I also recommend drying your feet thoroughly after bathing and wearing clean white socks until the fungus clears up. The dye in some dark socks can irritate the areas that are affected. If you need to wear dark socks, wear a pair of white socks underneath. Now, let me explain how to use this.

In this situation, the patient is asking for help and the pharmacist is clearly the expert. Therefore, advice giving is not only appropriate but helpful. By giving advice in a quiet and confident way, the pharmacist gains the patient's trust and makes the patient feel comfortable with asking questions in the future.

EXAMPLE 2

Patient: (30-year-old woman) I've been taking these birth control pills for three years now and my husband says I need to keep taking them. We don't want to have a baby yet, but I don't like the idea of taking something like this for so long. He wants me to because it's convenient for him. What do you think I should do?

Pharmacist: It's your body. If you don't want to take them, don't. He can't tell you what to do. He's your husband, not your boss.

There is truth in what the pharmacist says, but is saying it appropriate or wise? Who is the expert here? Clearly the patient is the expert (at least more so than the pharmacist) on her relationship with her husband. In this situation, we don't know the whole picture or all of the variables. We don't know for certain if her husband really said what she claims he did. It is possible that he did. It is also possible that the patient wants to be able to go home and tell her husband that the pharmacist said to stop taking the pill. The problem with the advice given here is that the pharmacist may not be prepared to deal with an angry husband when he comes into the pharmacy. Issues need to be sorted. The pharmacist could give expert counseling to both the husband and wife on different methods of birth control and relate to both of them the risks of the various methods. This would be appropriate and helpful. It is ultimately up to the couple to sort this out and decide which method is best for them. That is their decision, no one else's. If the patient wants to know what to do, the pharmacist can simply state that she would be happy to talk to the patient and her husband about the risks of long-term use and effectiveness of the pill and other methods of birth control, but that it is entirely up to her and her husband which method they choose.

Generalizing or Comparing

This type of response, like reassurance, is sometimes useful when patients are looking for a guarantee or wanting to feel less alone. However, it may not work in situations in which patients want to be understood and don't want their problems compared with anyone else's problems. Here are two examples:

EXAMPLE 1

Patient: Can you guarantee that this medicine is gonna keep me from having a stroke or heart attack?

Pharmacist: If you take this medicine the way you should, lower your salt intake and cholesterol, and get some exercise, I can guarantee that you will greatly reduce the risk of stroke or heart attack. This medicine has been shown to be very effective in treating high blood pressure if taken properly.

The patient wants a guarantee that he won't have a stroke or a heart attack if he takes the medicine. Although we cannot guarantee that that won't happen, we can speak generally about decreasing risk factors. Generalizing is effective in this situation.

EXAMPLE 2

Patient's father: My poor baby. She's really had a hard time with these ear infections. This is the second antibiotic in the last 3 months.

Pharmacist: (matter-of-factly) This seems to be the age for this. We see lots of kids with ear infections.

Patient's father: Is that supposed to make me feel better? My little girl is suffering.

Pharmacist: I'm sure she is.

Like reassurance, generalizing or comparing runs the risk of minimizing the problem in the eyes of the person presenting it. A way to avoid this is to respond empathically and wait and see if the patient asks for a comparison. That would indicate that reassurance is wanted, and the pharmacist could respond, "It certainly is distressing for both you and your baby when she gets an ear infection. It's a help-less feeling when kids are suffering" and then wait to see what direction the parent goes next. Like reassurance, comparisons and generalizations in such situations are often motivated by our own discomfort and usually are not helpful.

Assertive, Aggressive, and Nonassertive Responses

The basic idea behind assertiveness is respect for self and respect for others. In other words, all human life has value and should therefore be respected. Aggressive people respect themselves but not others, and nonassertive people respect others more than themselves. (See Chapter 6 for more on this topic.) Let's look at a dia-logue in which the pharmacist responds using assertiveness, aggressiveness, and nonassertiveness. In this situation, a patient claims for the third time that the phar-macist shorted her five tablets on her prescription.

Assertiveness

Patient: Oh, sir. (calling to the pharmacist and holding up her bottle) I just went out to my car with this, and you did it again. You shorted me five tablets.

Pharmacist: Mrs. Smith, I saw on your record that we had shorted you twice before, so I was very careful and counted your tablets twice today to make sure that the problem did not occur again.

Patient: Well, even so, it happened again. I'm five tablets short. You must have counted wrong. I'm supposed to have 50 tablets and there are only 45 here.

Pharmacist: I feel certain that I gave you 50 tablets. Therefore, I won't be giving you five more tablets today.

Patient: Well, you're wrong.

Pharmacist: (calmly) As I said, I was especially careful this time, so I won't be giving you five more tablets today.

Patient: This is ridiculous!

Pharmacist: (calmly) I understand your frustration.

Patient: Well, I just might have to take my business elsewhere.

Pharmacist: I hope you won't, but that certainly is up to you.

The pharmacist remains calm and acknowledges the patient's concerns but maintains his position. He does so in a way that shows respect for himself and the patient. Rather than caving in to manipulation, he allows the patient to choose what to do. The communication from the pharmacist is respectful, thoughtful, caring, and clear.

Aggressiveness

Patient: Oh, sir. (calling to the pharmacist and holding up her bottle) I just went out to my car with this, and you did it again. You shorted me five tablets.

Pharmacist: We're on to you, Mrs. Smith. We already went through this two other times with you, and it isn't going to happen again.

Patient: What are you talking about?

Pharmacist: We know your game. We're not going to give you extra tablets, so save your breath. We double-counted this time.

Patient: I've never been so insulted in all my life. I'll never come back here again.

Pharmacist: Fine.

This pharmacist is disrespectful to the patient. He is more interested in winning and in shaming the patient than in solving a problem. He attacks the patient, not the problem. Embarrassing her solves nothing. It is sad that some people use the injustices of others to justify their own bad behavior. The fact that Mrs. Smith is trying to get away with something does not mean that she has to be treated like a criminal.

Nonassertiveness

Patient: Oh, sir. (calling to the pharmacist and holding up her bottle) I just went out to my car with this, and you did it again. You shorted me five tablets.

Pharmacist: Oh, gosh, not again. I'm so sorry. I thought I got it right this time. I'll get you five more.

In this case, the pharmacist is afraid to assert that he has double-counted the tablets and is so afraid of upsetting the patient that he fails to respect himself. This gives the patient permission to continue her inappropriate behavior in the future.

Judging

The last response we will discuss is judging. There really isn't any benefit to this response, unless needing to be self-righteous is important. This response alienates people and shows a lack of understanding and a desire to be right rather than caring. Here's an example of judging.

Technician: I am so upset at Mrs. Brown. She is never nice to anyone when she comes in and never has anything pleasant to say. She criticizes everything.

Pharmacist: You obviously don't know how to handle Mrs. Brown. Don't take things so personally. You're overreacting.

Technician: Thanks a lot! Sorry I'm not as perfect as you!

The pharmacist does not listen to the technician's feelings. The technician is hurt and frustrated. The pharmacist could help the technician more by being understanding than by judging her behavior. Telling people they are overreacting is simply insensitive and a way to try to put them in their place. It is not at all caring. A more caring response would have been, "I know that you're very frustrated. Mrs. Brown really is difficult to deal with. She's a hard person to be around." This response has a higher probability of eliciting an inquiry from the technician about how the pharmacist handles Mrs. Brown. The previous response does not open up an opportunity for learning.

Summary

This chapter's discussion of types of responses and the examples given can assist you in choosing a response that is appropriate for the situation.

 Questions for Reflection

1. What is the difference between reassurance and empathy? A patient says, "I am so frightened. My doctor told me my diabetes is out of control." Respond with reassurance, and then respond with empathy.
2. When is it appropriate and inappropriate to give advice?
3. Distinguish between assertive, nonassertive, and aggressive responses.
4. Does empathy always work? Discuss when and why it does and when and why it doesn't.
5. When is it appropriate to use closed versus open-ended questions?

Reference

1. Dickson DA, Hargie O, Morrow NC. *Communication Skills Training for Health Professionals*. London: Chapman and Hall; 1989.

Chapter 12
PERSUASIVE COMMUNICATION

At one time or another, each of us has tried to persuade someone to do something. Most likely, we have met with varying degrees of success. Certain principles must be followed for persuasive communication to be effective, or it can backfire and cause more resistance

> **Persuasive communication is a conscious effort to influence the beliefs, attitudes, and, ultimately, the behaviors of another person.**

to engaging in the target behavior. Much research has been done on persuasive communication. In this chapter, persuasive strategies will be discussed and illustrated to help improve your powers of persuasion.

What Is Persuasive Communication?

Communication that is persuasive is directed toward changing or altering another person's beliefs, attitudes, and, ultimately, behaviors. According to Engel and colleagues,[1] attitudes have three components: *cognitive*—the manner in which the attitude object is perceived, *affective*—feelings of like or dislike toward the object, and *behavioral*—action tendencies toward the attitude object. The cognitive component is the person's belief about the attitude object. The idea is that beliefs affect attitudes, which affect behaviors: Change a person's beliefs or attitudes and you change the person's behaviors. Wouldn't it be wonderful if the world were that simple. Although beliefs, attitudes, and behaviors are related, the relationships are not always straightforward. A few examples will help clarify this.

Mrs. Jones is 80 years old. She knows that many people take medicines and that they get help from them. She, however, doesn't like to put any kind of medicine in her body. She believes that medicines can help other people, but she does not like (affective component) medicines, so she won't take them.

Mr. Smith thinks that Mercedes makes a great car (belief), and he really likes the way a Mercedes looks and performs (affective component). However, he isn't going to buy one because he can't afford it.

Heath Taylor, age 20, believes that medicines can really help people and has taken medicine for illnesses, but he has compliance problems because of his busy schedule.

These people all have positive beliefs about medications, but their attitudes and behaviors are different. Positive beliefs don't necessarily produce positive behaviors. For Mr. Smith, an intervening variable (money) precluded him from purchasing (the behavior) a Mercedes, even though he believes they are good cars and he likes them. Different strategies are needed to effect behavior change. One size does not fit all.

The terms *persuasion* and *influence* are often used interchangeably, but there is a distinction between the two. When someone is influenced by another, there is often a change in the person's beliefs, attitudes, or behavior; this sounds a lot like persuasion. However, we can influence people without consciously attempting to do so.[2] For example, as a parent, I could positively (or negatively) influence the behavior of my child by the way I interact with others. I may not be consciously aware that my child is watching and learning, but the influence is there nonetheless. Persuasion, on the other hand, is conscious. There is a volitional attempt to influence someone else.

Influences on Persuasive Messages

Many factors determine the effectiveness of a persuasive message. Four major factors are (1) the message source, (2) believability of the message, (3) environmental factors, and (4) comprehension and retention of the message. These factors overlap a great deal. Certainly, the credibility of the message source influences the believability of the message, and comprehension and retention of the message are also influenced by the believability of the message.

Message source. For a persuasive message to have its intended impact, the message source (the pharmacist) must be seen as credible. Credibility involves recognized expertise and the desire to do what is right, serve the patient, be warm, and be fair. Expertise alone is not enough. The patient must perceive that the pharmacist's expert power is being used not to manipulate or control, but to do what is best for the patient. Of course, this involves finding out what the patient thinks is best, too. It is important to note that expertise is not ascribed to a pharmacist simply because of a societal role. It must be demonstrated in a way that supports the patient. Expertise that "puts the patient in his place" is not generally persuasive. A few examples will illustrate this point.

Mrs. Jones enters the pharmacy to have her antihypertensive medication refilled.

Pharmacist: Hello, Mrs. Jones. How are you today?

Mrs. Jones: Just fine. Couldn't be better.

Pharmacist: Great! I'll go refill your prescription.

Pharmacist: (a few moments later) Mrs. Jones, I noticed that your blood pressure medicine should have run out several weeks ago. Are you taking your medicine the way you're supposed to take it?

Mrs. Jones: Oh sure, every time I get a headache.

Pharmacist: That doesn't make any sense. How often is that?

Mrs. Jones: Oh, maybe once a week.

Pharmacist: Mrs. Jones, that's not how you're supposed to take it at all. Where did you get such an idea? Didn't you read the label instructions? It says take it every day.

Mrs. Jones: What's your problem? Just give me my medicine! (grabs the bag) Put it on my account. (exits the pharmacy)

Pharmacist: But you're not taking it the right way.

The pharmacist is in no position to have influence here because of the approach he takes. He will probably have to call Mrs. Jones later and get this situation straightened out. Rather than taking a calm approach, he berates Mrs. Jones. She is unwilling to listen and leaves without finding out what the problem is. Let's see how this might have been approached:

Pharmacist: Hello, Mrs. Jones. How are you today?

Mrs. Jones: Just fine. Couldn't be better.

Pharmacist: Great! I'll go refill your prescription.

Pharmacist: (a few moments later) Mrs. Jones, I noticed that your blood pressure medicine should have run out several weeks ago. Can you tell me how you're taking it?

Mrs. Jones: Oh sure, every time I get a headache.

Pharmacist: (calmly) So you take it when you get a headache because you believe that you have headaches when your blood pressure is up?

Mrs. Jones: Exactly!

Pharmacist: That makes sense. However, we should have done a better job of explaining to you how to take this medicine.

Mrs. Jones: What do you mean?

Pharmacist: It is certainly true that people with high blood pressure sometimes get headaches. But it is usually stress, not your high blood pressure, that is causing them. It is really very difficult, if not impossible, to tell when your blood pressure is up without measuring it. The medicine should be taken once a day for you to get the most benefit from it.

Mrs. Jones: Once a day? I didn't know that.

Pharmacist: Well, let's have you start taking it once a day from now on, even if you don't have a headache. I want to make sure your blood pressure stays controlled.

Mrs. Jones: So do I. I never knew.

Pharmacist: I know. Again, I sure can understand the confusion.

This pharmacist took responsibility, and, because he did not blame or berate the patient, she was willing to listen. She was able to be influenced because she felt understood. The pharmacist's communication was directed toward solving a problem, not ascribing blame. Even though he knew the label directions were not being followed, he felt no need to point this out and risk embarrassing her.

There is a great deal of literature indicating that men and women use different persuasive strategies. However, the literature is inconsistent about exactly what those differences in persuasive communication strategies are and whether they result from gender differences or differences in roles. For example, some literature reports that women use a more democratic and participative leadership style to have influence, whereas men tend to be more autocratic and directive.[3] Other research attributes these differences more to role in the organization than to gender. That is, as women move higher in the organization, their communication tends to be more autocratic and directive.

Regardless, Gilligan and Attanucci[4] found that "men employ a 'justice' orientation in reasoning about moral choices by emphasizing the importance of rights, respect, and impartiality, whereas women employ a 'care' orientation in their moral reasoning by emphasizing mutual participation, cooperation, and attention to individuals' feelings and needs." Men are most likely to influence by focusing on rights and responsibilities, and women are likely to influence by emphasizing issues relating to feelings and caring.[5] These influence focuses are not right or wrong, they are simply the way many men and women attempt to influence others. These strategies do work, but only for individuals who orient in the same way. Both men and women need to be flexible enough to realize that appeals to justice also work for many women and appeals to emotions and caring also work for many men. A flexible set of influence strategies is needed.

Believability of the message. The believability of the message is related not only to the credibility of the message source but also to whether the message fits the patient's belief system. Some patients may find it very hard to believe (and understand) concepts that we take for granted. For example, potency is often a difficult concept for patients. A patient may have been taking a tablet for pain relief. This tablet was taken twice a day and was quite large, but the patient got no relief despite the fact that he was taking it properly. The physician then prescribed another medication that is more potent, is taken less often, and comes in much smaller tablets. It may be difficult for some patients to accept that this smaller tablet is going to help if the larger one taken twice as often did not help. As a result, the patient may not even try the new medicine unless he is persuaded by the pharmacist. To be persuasive, the pharmacist will first have to acknowledge and objectively reflect back an understanding of the patient's beliefs. Then, factual information about potency will have to be given that makes sense to the patient. Analogies may need to be used to allow the patient to understand the concept of potency. One analogy that might make sense to a patient is that of black pepper versus cayenne pepper, the idea being that smaller amounts of cayenne pepper have more potent effects in the mouth than larger amounts of black pepper.

Another issue that may be difficult to grasp is that many drugs have multiple indications at various dosing schedules. For example, diazepam can be used for anxiety, epilepsy, and muscle relaxation. It is often very difficult for patients to understand how this can occur. Therefore, when a patient asks, "What's this medicine for?" the best answer is, "Could you tell me what caused you to see the doctor?" rather than, "It's for numerous things, like anxiety, epilepsy, and muscle relaxation."

Environmental factors. Environmental factors in a pharmacy include privacy, noise, interruptions, and distractions that can affect whether a message is heard and understood. It is important that persuasive messages be delivered in an environment that, to the extent possible, is free from noise, distractions, and interruptions. Each time these things occur, the likelihood of message comprehension and retention decreases. The pharmacist should do as much as possible to create private areas for talking with patients. If this is not possible, then attempts should be made to pull patients away from sources of noise, interruptions, and distractions.

Comprehension and retention of the message. Obviously, for a persuasive message to be effective it must be understood and recalled. We have already discussed the effects of environmental factors on comprehension and recall. In addition, as one might suspect, the credibility of the message source is a critical variable in comprehension and recall. I probably won't listen to the message if I don't believe that you are a credible source or if I question the believability of the message.

Another key factor that affects comprehension is the language level of the message. Is the message conveyed in language that is understood by the receiver? Too often in health care, providers use jargon that is common to medicine and pharmacy but not to patients. For example, a 67-year-old woman came into a pharmacy and asked a pharmacist how her methyldopa lowered her blood pressure. She was told that it was a dopa decarboxylase inhibitor. (I wish I could say that I made this up, but it is a true story.) The woman looked confused, but she said, "Oh, OK," and then left the pharmacy. I'm sure that she found the message believable. I'm not so sure she understood a word the pharmacist said. It is vitally important to use language the patient can understand. It is better to say "high blood pressure" than "hypertension."

Another comprehension problem has to do with the receiver's interpretation of the message. Sometimes, our communication with patients seems clear to us but is open to interpretation by the patient. For example, we know that when we tell patients to "take one tablet twice a day" we mean that we want them to take a tablet approximately every 12 hours. But if this meaning is not made explicit, problems may occur. How is the direction to "take one tablet after meals and at bedtime" interpreted? It depends on how many meals you eat a day. A patient with diabetes may eat six or seven small meals each day and take seven or eight tablets. I eat two meals a day, so I would take three tablets. If neither of these responses is correct, then we need to be much more explicit in our directions.

Finally, the only way to know whether a message is understood and can be recalled is to ask patients to repeat back their understanding of the message. This can be done by simply saying, "Just to be sure that I wasn't unclear about what I told you, can you please tell me how you are going to take your medicine?"

Direct Persuasive Strategies

We have discussed factors affecting persuasive communication and stated that persuasive communication is a conscious effort to influence the beliefs, attitudes, and, ultimately, the behaviors of another person. We now turn to persuasive strategies. The following paragraphs discuss direct persuasive strategies.

Consciousness-raising. Consciousness-raising in the pharmacist–patient relationship involves either providing information about the patient's illness and treatment in a straightforward, objective way or helping the patient become more aware of healthy or unhealthy behaviors (or beliefs or attitudes) in which he or she is currently engaged. Regardless, having influence is the objective. Providing information seems straightforward, but the way we communicate information can either result in clarity or cause confusion. The language we use must be clear and understandable. Helping the patient become more aware of healthy or unhealthy behaviors is less straightforward, as the following example shows.

Pharmacist: Mr. Johnson, I am concerned about the fact that you continue to smoke even though you have asthma.

Patient: I feel OK.

Pharmacist: That's great. I hope you do. Over time, cigarette smoking will continue to damage your lungs, and your breathing will become more and more difficult. I would hate for you to have to go to the emergency room or be hospitalized. Also, smoking puts you at greater risk for other illnesses.

Patient: I didn't know asthma was that serious.

Pharmacist: It can be if it's not controlled, and it's almost impossible to control if you continue to smoke. That concerns me a great deal.

Patient: I need to give this some serious thought.

Pharmacist: I know of several products and smoking cessation programs that are helpful. Give me a call when you're ready.

The pharmacist confronted the patient about his smoking and used consciousness-raising to address the problem directly. The pharmacist was able to have influence on the patient's beliefs because he was objective and demonstrated caring.

Messages that arouse fear. There is research supporting the idea that a message can be persuasive if it arouses fear. The idea is that avoiding problems is rewarding. According to Stubblefield,[6] "Messages that arouse fear can promote health behavior change if they meet the following conditions: (1) the message provides a strong argument that the recipient will suffer a negative consequence if the recommendations are not accepted; and (2) the message provides strong assurance that adoption of the recommendations will eliminate the negative consequences." Two studies evaluated the effects of fear-arousing health messages in women. One involved cancer in general and the involved other breast cancer and breast self-examination. The fear-arousal messages did increase participation in preventive measures.[6] After hearing a fear-arousal message, the patient must believe that his or her actions will lead to a reduction of the threat. Let's see how this might work.

Pharmacist: Mrs. Ackerman, I am quite concerned that you are taking only about 30% of your doses for your high blood pressure. Given that your blood pressure is 170/110, I am very concerned about your having a stroke or heart attack.

Patient: Don't you think you're overreacting? I feel just fine.

Pharmacist: That's part of the problem. People can't tell when their blood pressure is up by how they feel. Most patients feel just fine even when their blood pressure is dangerously high. You are still putting a strain on your heart. It is very important that you take your medicine every day as prescribed to get your blood pressure down and reduce your risk of a stroke or a heart attack.

Patient: Can you guarantee that that will keep me from having a heart attack?

Pharmacist: I can guarantee that you will greatly reduce your risks and that you are asking for trouble if you don't take your medicine as prescribed, each day. Is remembering to take it once a day a problem for you?

Patient: Not really. I just didn't know I was at such high risk.

Pharmacist: This is really very important.

Patient: OK.

Pharmacist: Please let me know if you have any problems.

This pharmacist used a fear-arousing appeal. It worked because the pharmacist expressed caring and concern, because the patient finally understands that she really is at risk, and because she believes that she can do what is necessary to reduce the risk.

Use of vivid information. Particularly in fear-arousal appeals, research supports the use of vivid rather than abstract information.[7] Vivid information includes emotional appeals and examples that the patient can relate to, such as examples of people (famous or otherwise) the patient's age. A concrete example helps make abstract information more real to the patient. In the above example of the patient with hypertension, pointing out that another patient recently had a stroke because of uncontrolled blood pressure (without mentioning the patient's name) could help this patient understand the problem more clearly.

In general, the research on negatively framed appeals (fear arousal) versus positively framed appeals has supported negative appeals in promoting health behaviors to avoid risk, such as the risk of cancer or osteoporosis.[6] More research is needed to evaluate these findings. Telling patients the benefits of taking their medicine properly and engaging in healthy behaviors is also vitally important.

Linguistic binds. One last category of direct persuasive appeals will be discussed—with caution. Linguistic binds are discussed in the persuasion literature and could have relevance to pharmacy practice. However, there is an element of deception in the use of linguistic binds. "Binds create the illusion of choice by using language that 'normally' offers a choice, where either choice you choose, you still go along with what the speaker wants."[8] Using linguistic binds causes one to walk a fine line between influence and manipulation. Here's an example of two linguistic binds:

Pharmacist: Mrs. Smith, I note from this new prescription that you are newly diagnosed with high blood pressure.

Patient: Yes, I just came from the doctor.

Pharmacist: The medicine the doctor prescribed is very effective if taken correctly.

Patient: Oh, believe me, I'll take it correctly. I don't want to have a stroke.

Pharmacist: Great! Dr. Stevens probably told you that the only way we can really know if your blood pressure is being controlled is to take regular readings using a blood pressure cuff.

Patient: Yes, he did say I should take my medicine even if I feel fine.

Pharmacist: Good. Since you will only be seeing Dr. Stevens every 3 months, I would like to either show you a blood pressure cuff for home use or offer a monitoring service that costs $30 per month for unlimited readings that I will fax to your doctor every 2 weeks. Which would you prefer?

Patient: Uh, I guess I would rather have the monitoring service.

Pharmacist: Great. Would you like to go ahead and set up your first appointment now, or when's a good time for you to meet to take your blood pressure? (Pharmacist has pen in hand to jot down a time.)

Patient: I guess Friday mornings.

Pharmacist: Good. 10 am this Friday?

Patient: OK.

Several issues need to be discussed here. First, offering to sell a blood pressure cuff or a monitoring service certainly is appropriate for any patient with high blood pressure. If patients with high blood pressure regularly had their blood pressure monitored, far fewer strokes or heart attacks might occur. Both times that the pharmacist uses the linguistic bind, the illusion of choice is presented. In the first bind, the pharmacist wants to sell a product or a service, either of which would benefit the patient and the pharmacist. The choice that's left out is to buy neither. In the second bind, the illusion of choice is setting up the first appointment. It's hard to argue against monitoring high blood pressure. It is a good thing for the patient to do. However, what concerns people about linguistic binds is the element of confusion or deception created. It seems not quite honest. Here, the expertise, authority, and power the pharmacist has is being used to force a choice. The linguistic binds are being used to benefit the patient and the pharmacist. Binds that benefit only the pharmacist at the expense of the patient are not appropriate and are ethically questionable.

When Direct Persuasive Attempts Fail

Even when all of the above guidelines are followed, there are times when persuasive strategies don't work or aren't very effective. When people strongly resist change, direct persuasive strategies are usually ineffective. These direct strategies often take the form of advice giving or "yes, but…" communication. Here's an example:

Pharmacist: Mr. Johnson, since you have asthma, you really need to quit smoking.

Mr. Johnson: (yes, but) I'm really not ready to quit. I like it too much. It relaxes me.

Pharmacist: (yes, but) Don't you think your health is important?

Mr. Johnson: (yes, but) Why don't you let me worry about that?

Pharmacist: (yes, but) I don't think you understand how serious this is.

Mr. Johnson: (yes, but) I don't think you understand how serious I am!

> Certain principles must be followed for persuasive communication to be effective, or it can backfire and cause more resistance to engaging in the target behavior.

This could go on and on—and usually does. The "yes, buts" actually force the patient to defend the very behavior you are trying to change. Remember, persuasion involves a conscious attempt to *influence*, not an attempt to *coerce or convince*. To influence people, it is especially important that they feel they are not being coerced or manipulated and that they have choices. Otherwise, people—especially resistant people—dig in further. The work of Miller and Rollnick[9] and Prochaska and colleagues[10] has added much to our understanding of patient resistance. Ambivalence is often the cause of such resistance.[9] When people are ambivalent, they often do nothing. Therefore, one approach is to provide objective, nonjudgmental information. If the patient is informed but is not ready to change because he or she is ambivalent about the ability to make the necessary changes, different strategies are needed.

One influence strategy involves attempting to see the world as the patient sees it and then clearly defining the choices that need to be made. Here's an example.

Pharmacist: Because of your asthma, I'm very concerned about your continuing to smoke.

Patient: I'm just not ready to quit. It really relaxes me.

Pharmacist: It would be hard to give up something that's relaxing.

Patient: Yeah, no kidding. You ever tried to quit smoking?

Pharmacist: No, but I know it's very hard for most people. I wanted you to know that I am concerned because smoking can make your asthma much worse. I do have some smoking cessation products that could help when you are ready to quit. The choice really is up to you.

Patient: I appreciate that. I'm just not ready.

Pharmacist: I understand. If you haven't had a chest X-ray lately, you might consider that just to make sure everything is OK. At least it would give you additional information for making an informed decision. Let me go ahead and show you how this asthma inhaler works.

This pharmacist was informative but did not try to coerce the patient into quitting. We cannot make people change their behavior. The pharmacist opened a door for future conversation and kept it open by nonjudgmentally directing his communication at what was appropriate for this patient.

Another strategy that often works for resistant patients involves self-persuasion and the use of cognitive dissonance. Cognitive dissonance theory states that a feeling of dissonance or distress occurs in people when they do or say something that runs in direct opposition to their beliefs or their self-concept. To reduce the dissonance produced, people will "try to bring those disparate cognitions into greater harmony."[11] It has been found that dissonance is very self-motivating. Therefore, if we can create dissonance in our communication with another, this will stimulate individuals to persuade themselves to do something to reduce the dissonance. Here are two examples of how this might work:

EXAMPLE 1

Patient: I'm just not ready to quit smoking. I find it very relaxing.

Pharmacist: What would you tell your teenage daughter, Sara, about smoking?

Patient: I'd tell her not to do it.

Pharmacist: Because?

Patient: For obvious health reasons, cost, and the like.

Pharmacist: Your smoking and the advice you would give seem a little inconsistent.

Patient: I suppose they are.

EXAMPLE 2

Patient: I'm just not ready to quit smoking. I find it very relaxing.

Pharmacist: It would be hard to give up something you find relaxing. What else do you like about smoking?

Patient: It gives me something to do with my hands, and I especially like lighting up after a meal. It's very relaxing. It also helps me keep weight off.

Pharmacist: Those things are important. Do you see any downside to smoking?

Patient: Oh sure, the usual health reasons, plus my wife says my breath and clothes smell. And it's become more and more expensive.

Pharmacist: So on the one hand, smoking relaxes you, gives you something to do with your hands, and keeps you from gaining weight, but on the other hand you realize that it is very bad for your health, your wife says your breath and clothes smell, and it's expensive.

Patient: Right.

Pharmacist: I did want you to know that I am concerned about your smoking, but I won't bug you about it. I do have some things that can help you stop if you get to that point.

In example 1, the pharmacist creates dissonance by creating a discrepancy between the patient's beliefs or values and what he actually does. In example 2, the dissonance is created by repeating back what the patient says is positive and negative about smoking. The dissonance becomes the stimulus for change. In both examples, the pharmacist is nonjudgmental and does not attempt to move the patient along too quickly—which would only create more resistance (see Chapter 8).

Summary

This chapter has described general principles of persuasive communication. In addition, direct and indirect examples of persuasive communication have been explored. The use of influence strategies that benefit the patient and enhance patient care has been emphasized. The reader is encouraged to try out several of these strategies, because patients respond to different forms of influence.

Questions for Reflection

1. What are linguistic binds? How can they be used effectively in pharmacy? What is the possible downside to them?
2. If the message source is an important element in the persuasiveness or believability of a message, what can pharmacists do to be seen as a more credible message source? What can a pharmacist do to make a message more believable to the patient?
3. Discuss various ways that a pharmacist could use consciousness-raising to improve adherence to a treatment plan.
4. Discuss the ways in which you can be more persuasive in your communication. What would you need to change or work on?
5. Why and under what conditions does persuasive communication cause more resistance rather than less?

References

1. Engel JF, Kollat DT, Blackwell RD. *Consumer Behavior*. 2nd ed. Hinsdale, Ill: Dryden Press; 1973.
2. McCroskey JC, Richmond VP, Stewart RA. *One on One: The Foundations of Interpersonal Communication*. Englewood Cliffs, NJ: Prentice Hall; 1986.
3. Baker MA. Gender and verbal communication in professional settings: a review of research. *Manag Commun Q*. 1991;5:36–63.
4. Gilligan C, Attanucci J. Two moral orientations: gender differences and similarities. *Merrill-Palmer Q*. 1988;34:223–37.
5. Kline SL. Gender issues in persuasive messages practices. *Womens Stud Commun*. 1998;4:68–88.
6. Stubblefield C. Persuasive communication: marketing health promotion. *Nurs Outlook*. 1997;45:173–7.
7. Rook KS. Encouraging preventive behavior for distant and proximal health threats: effects of vivid versus abstract information. *J Gerontol*. 1986;41:526–34.
8. Cleveland KE. How to use linguistic binds to persuade. Available at http://pertinent.com/pertinfo/business/kenrickP4.html. Accessed March 2000.
9. Miller WR, Rollnick S. *Motivational Interviewing*. New York: Guilford Press; 1991.
10. Prochaska JO, DiClemente CC. *The Transtheoretical Approach: Crossing Traditional Boundaries of Therapy*. Homewood, Ill: Dow Jones-Irwin; 1984.
11. Aronson E. The power of self-persuasion. *Am Psychol*. 1999;11:875–84.

Chapter 13
IMMEDIACY: HOW WORD CHOICE AND NONVERBAL CUES AFFECT THE RELATIONSHIP[a]

In this chapter we will examine how the words we choose influence the nature and quality of pharmacists' relationships with their patients. We will then examine how nonverbal cues can enhance or detract from the quality of pharmacist–patient therapeutic relationships.

By listening carefully to the way people say things, we can quickly recognize that a speaker's choice of words reveals a wealth of information about the speaker's true feelings or attitudes toward a topic, event, or person. Even when speakers skillfully try to disguise their feelings and emotions, particular attention to the speaker's word choice can reveal true intentions or motivations. This chapter will describe principles that pharmacists can use to make inferences about patients' feelings or attitudes toward a topic, event, or person. Equally important, the chapter will provide principles pharmacists can use to craft more efficient and effective messages for their patients.

Verbal Immediacy

In 1968, Wiener and Mehrabian[1] described verbal immediacy as a model of communication that analyzes variations in word use as a basis for inferring different feelings or attitudes of the speaker. For example, a pharmacist could say, "You and I should discuss your options" or "We should discuss your options."

> Verbal immediacy refers to the degree of separation created between the speaker and the object of the speaker's communication as a result of the particular words used by the speaker.

Through careful examination of messages that appear to say the same thing, but with different words, we can infer different feelings or attitudes on the part of the speaker. The variations in word choice indicate different degrees of separation from the object of the speaker's communication. "You and I" may be equivalent in meaning to "we," but the "we" statement represents more immediate communication than the "you and I" statement. The "you and I" statement is an example of nonimmediacy. It is considered nonimmediate because it uses two symbols ("you" and "I") to designate two separate entities when the language provides the option of using only one symbol ("we").

---

[a]This chapter was written with the invaluable assistance of Amanda K. Diggs, PhD, Assistant Professor, Troy State University, Montgomery, Alabama.

Nonimmediate	Immediate
You and I	We

Verbal immediacy refers to the degree of separation created between the speaker and the object of the speaker's communication as a result of the particular words used by the speaker. Inferences can be drawn about speakers' feelings concerning things they are communicating about, their communication, or the listeners.

Why Do We Use Nonimmediate Language?

Wiener and Mehrabian use the term nonimmediacy to refer to "any indication of separation, nonidentity, attenuation of directness, or change in intensity of interaction" among the communicator, the listener, the object of communication, or the communication itself. Nonimmediacy represents a speaker's attempt to separate himself or herself from the object of the communication, from the listener, or from the communication. This separation can be construed to represent avoidance behavior motivated by a negative emotional state toward the object, listener, or communication. In other words, nonimmediacy represents an individual's attempt to avoid identifying with unpleasant objects, persons, or topics. Nonimmediacy is a technique for distancing yourself from objects, events, persons, or topics that you'd rather avoid.

Often, feelings and emotions cannot be easily expressed in words. In fact, in most cultures restraints are imposed on communication regarding emotion, evaluation, or preference in general.[2] This is true particularly concerning the expression of negative feelings and emotions, evaluation, or preference.

Nonimmediacy and the Health Care Provider

Von Friederichs-Fitzwater[3] studied the use of verbally immediate language in conversations between health care providers and terminally ill patients. Von Friederichs-Fitzwater's review of the literature revealed that health care providers are uncomfortable when communicating with dying patients.[3] Furthermore, health care providers are uncomfortable discussing the topics of death and dying.

That analysis showed that health care providers used far more nonimmediate language than the dying patients they cared for. This is evidence that communicating with dying patients represents an essential but difficult task for health care professionals. The study showed that dying patients did use some nonimmediate language in their communications with health care providers. Like health care providers, patients use nonimmediate language as a means of dealing with uncomfortable feelings.

The researcher suggested that patients' use of nonimmediate language may be con-nected to their fears of abandonment, pain, loss of independence, or fear of the un-known. This further suggests that patients and health care providers may choose to use more nonimmediate language in an effort to protect feelings of vulnerability, guilt, or resentment.

In that study, the differences between the verbal immediacy scores of physi-cians, nurses, and hospice workers were not significant. This suggests that hospice workers and nurses are as uncomfortable as physicians in communicating with dy-ing patients. Perhaps all the health care providers included in the study used nonimmediacy or distancing behavior as a means of coping with such an emotion-ally taxing situation as death and dying.

Implications for Pharmacists

Sometimes, health care providers' communication with patients is marked by a climate of distance and aloofness. Like other health care professionals, pharmacists may be using nonimmediate language when communicating with particular pa-tients or when discussing difficult or unpleasant topics, issues, or events. The use of nonimmediate language may hamper the establishment of healthy, trusting thera-peutic relationships with patients. In addition, the use of nonimmediate language may prove detrimental when trying to build rapport with patients.

Pharmacists should consider adopting a more immediate style of communication. They should use more immediate language to help build therapeutic relationships with patients. Pharmacists are in a unique position to be the health care providers who create environments where patients feel comfortable enough to communicate openly and honestly about their health-related concerns and issues. This niche is currently unfilled by other health care providers.

Steps to More Immediate Language

Step 1a: Identify topics and issues that make you uncomfortable. Make a list of topics, issues, objects, and events that you find difficult to discuss or that make you uncomfortable. Here are some examples: death and dying, cancer, AIDS, sexual dysfunction. You should be more specific in your list.

Step 1b: Identify groups and persons with whom you feel uncomfortable. Make a list of groups and individuals who make you feel uncomfortable and with whom you find it difficult to communicate. Again, be more specific than the following examples: minority groups, mentally challenged people, physically challenged people, people suffering from specific diseases.

Step 2: Identify nonimmediate language when it is spoken. Wiener and Mehrabian devised six categories for identifying nonimmediate language. This chapter outlines three very basic categories for identifying nonimmediate language (symbol used, us versus them, and temporal). Remember that nonimmediate language works to separate the speaker from the listener or from the object or subject spoken about. Nonimmediacy serves as a means of exclusion rather than inclusion. Therefore, nonimmediate language hinders rapport building, because it excludes either the pharmacist or the patient. Exclusive communication reveals negative feelings and emotions and alludes to treatment that is not personal.

Symbol used. The "symbol used" category of nonimmediacy examines the symbols that take the place of the referent or word and the adjectives used to describe words. The more ambiguous or nonspecific the symbols used, the more nonimmediate the language.

Notice the words you use as symbols for people, places, objects, events, and so on. For example, when referring to Mrs. Henderson, you may select the symbol "my patient," "a patient," or "the person"—in decreasing degrees of immediacy. The final symbol, "the per-

> The use of nonimmediate language may hamper the establishment of healthy, trusting therapeutic relationships with patients.

son," represents the greatest degree of separation of the pharmacist from the patient. It expresses the most negative degree of emotion and feeling about Mrs. Henderson.

The symbols for people, objects, and events being communicated are often pronouns. The less specific the symbol, the more nonimmediate the communication. For example, if the pharmacist asks why the patient smokes, the patient might give the following responses:

I smoke because I enjoy it. (most immediate)
We smoke because we enjoy it.
One smokes because one enjoys it.
You (you meaning I) smoke because you enjoy it. (least immediate)

The patient's increasing nonimmediacy is a means of separating himself from the subject of the communication. The symbols become less and less specific.

In another example, a pharmacist might respond, regarding a pharmacy convention that he or she attended:

I discussed the new legislation. (most immediate)
We discussed the new legislation.
Pharmacists discussed the new legislation.
There was a discussion of the new legislation. (least immediate)

Or, a pharmacist might say to a patient:

Remember, we said that you should come in for a checkup. (most immediate)
Remember, you said that you would come in for a checkup.
Remember, it was said that you should come in for a checkup. (least immediate)

When you substitute words such as "everyone" for "I," you indicate nonimmediacy and nonidentity with the object of the communication. In such instances, the speaker works to exclude himself or herself from the object or subject of the communication. For example, a pharmacist says, "Mrs. Jones, I noticed that you're 5 days late on your blood pressure medicine." The patient replies:

I forget to take my medication sometimes. (most immediate)
Everyone forgets to take their medications sometimes. (least immediate)

To assess the immediacy of your use of symbols in communication with patients, answer the question, Do I include or exclude myself when I communicate with patients? For example:

Am I more likely to refer to a patient as "my patient" or "the patient"?

When talking about a patient's problem(s), am I more likely to refer to the patient's problem as "my problem," "our problem," "your problem," or "their problem"?

The terms "my" and "our" are considered more immediate than "your" or "their." Use of the terms "my" and "our" includes, rather than excludes, the pharmacist. By using "my" or "our" in discussing a patient's problem, the pharmacist takes responsibility and participates in the process with the patient. This can be very effective in building rapport. The use of these terms indicates to the patient that he or she does not have to deal with the problem alone. Rather, the patient can infer that he or she has a partner.

On the other hand, use of the terms "your" and "their" excludes the pharmacist from the problem. Using "your problem" or "their problem" separates the pharmacist from the problem. Patients can infer that they must deal with the problem alone.

When discussing a patient's options, are you more likely to say, "You and I should discuss your options" or "We should discuss your options"? "You and I" represents more nonimmediate language than "we." "We" represents more inclusive communication than "you and I." Using "you and I" signifies the pharmacist's attempt to separate himself or herself from the patient.

Nonimmediate	Immediate
Your, yours	My, mine
Their, theirs	Our, ours
You and I	We
He or she and I	We

Us versus them. The "us versus them" category of nonimmediacy describes the relationship between the communicator and the object of the communication in terms of space and time (here and now versus far away and long ago). Words denoting time and space clearly identify the degree of separation between the communicator and the object.

To assess your use of these indicators of nonimmediacy, ask yourself, Do I try to include my patients or exclude them in my communication endeavors? The first step in identifying nonimmediate language in this category is to notice when you use the term "that" as opposed to "this," or "those" as opposed to "these."

For example, the pharmacist says, "I don't understand those people" or "when those people are in the same room." "Those" is considered nonimmediate because it signifies separation between the speaker and the object of the communication. The use of the word "those" as opposed to "these" may be interpreted as signifying the speaker's negative emotions, evaluations, or lack of personal feelings about "those" people.

Nonimmediate	Immediate
The	My
	Your
That	This
Those	These
They	
Them	

Temporal. The temporal category of nonimmediacy describes the relationship between the speaker and the object of the communication in terms of time. The speaker separates himself or herself from the object of communication by using language that refers to the past or future as opposed to the present. Note your use of adverbial clauses introduced by "when," "during," or "while." For example, the pharmacist might say:

Do you feel offended *when people talk about your cancer?* (least immediate)
Would you feel offended if we talked about your cancer? (more immediate)

Do you feel embarrassed *while receiving information about your birth control?* (least immediate)
Would discussing your birth control prescription with me embarrass you? (more immediate)

During your visits with me, can you and I begin to discuss your concerns about your disease? (least immediate)
Can we begin to discuss concerns you may have about this disease? (more immediate)

Step 3: Identify when and with whom you use nonimmediate language. As in step 1, make lists: I do this when rushed, stressed, anxious or nervous, irritated, frightened, uncertain. I do this with Mrs. Peach (she's mean and unpleasant), Mr. Doe (he has severe facial burns and his appearance frightens me), Mr. X (he cross-dresses, and I can't remember whether I should refer to him as he or she), unwed mothers who continue to have child after child after child, "aristocrats" who think I should show them preferential treatment and stop whatever I'm doing to take care of their needs immediately.

Pulling It Together

To summarize, here is a nonimmediate dialogue, followed by a more immediate dialogue, between a pharmacist and patient. The focus is on the pharmacist's verbal immediacy.

Nonimmediate Language

Pharmacist: What can we do for you today, Mrs. Edwards?

Patient: I can't believe the doctor put me on insulin injections for my diabetes.

Pharmacist: Well, you know, <u>a lot of patients with diabetes</u> take insulin injections.

Patient: But I hate needles.

Pharmacist: <u>Most patients with diabetes</u> say they don't give them a second thought once they get used to them.

Patient: Well, (sigh) I don't like them.

Pharmacist: Don't worry. <u>Everyone</u> who takes shots does just fine eventually. You'll do just fine.

This dialogue is a prime example of nonimmediacy. The whole tone of this interaction is one of nonidentity and detachment. First, the pharmacist distances himself from the patient's problem. He does not address Mrs. Edwards's concerns. Not once during the interaction does the pharmacist appear to identify with the patient's emotional state. Second, the pharmacist does not deal with the patient on a personal level. Notice how the pharmacist talks about other patients instead of Mrs. Edwards as an individual.

Immediate Language

Pharmacist: Hi, Mrs. Edwards. What can I do for you today?

Patient: I can't believe the doctor put me on insulin injections for my diabetes.

Pharmacist: I see (looking at the prescription). You are obviously very concerned about this. Do needles scare you?

Patient: Yes, they do.

Pharmacist: Mrs. Edwards, did the doctor show you how to give yourself an injection?

Patient: No.

Pharmacist: Well, <u>I'd</u> like to show you how to safely and properly administer the injections. <u>Soon</u>, you'll be doing this like a pro. I think that might help with some of the fear.

Patient: Well, (sigh) I don't know.

Pharmacist: Mrs. Edwards, <u>I'll</u> help you any way <u>I</u> can. <u>If we work together</u>, I know you can do this.

This dialogue is an example of immediacy. First, the pharmacist does not distance himself from the patient's problem. He addresses Mrs. Edwards's concerns. Notice how this pharmacist uses a lot of "I" statements in regard to helping the patient. Second, the pharmacist deals with the patient on a personal level. The pharmacist does not make references to other patients, but talks about how Mrs. Edwards sees the problem. Note how much more personal this pharmacist's language is.

Summary of Verbal Immediacy

Using more verbally immediate language is one way of building rapport with patients. By using more verbally immediate language, pharmacists begin the process of identifying with their patients and their patients' problems. Furthermore, using more verbally immediate language can be instrumental in establishing relationships with patients based on a teamwork approach to managing their illnesses.

Nonverbal Immediacy

We have seen how the words we choose can serve to create either emotional distance or immediacy. Now we will discuss nonverbal communication. Recent literature suggests that nonverbal immediacy behaviors on the part of physicians and other health care providers are very much related to patient satisfaction with care, and hence, outcomes.[4]

What Is Nonverbal Communication?

Nonverbal communication includes the way space or physical distance is used in communication (*proxemics*), the use of time in our communication (*chronemics*), the amount of eye contact or gaze (*oculesics*), the use of touch (*haptics*), body movement (*kinesics*), the use and choice of objects in communication, such as clothing or symbols (*objectics*), and the use and quality of the human voice, such as changes in tone and pitch (*vocalics*). An estimated 55% of the meaning we derive in the communication process is the direct result of nonverbal messages, approximately 38% comes from vocal cues, and 7% comes from the verbal messages.[5] This has very important implications for communicating with patients. We often focus on the words spoken, but 93% of the meaning of a message is derived from nonverbal cues. It is very important that there is congruence between verbal and nonverbal cues. Let's look at each of the nonverbal areas and see how they might affect our communication with patients. The assumption is that we want our communication to be more, rather than less, immediate. That is, we want our communication to cause us to be perceived as warm, caring, and approachable.

Proxemics

Proxemics is concerned with the physical distance between people when they communicate. Different types of communication require different spacing. For example, a person giving a public speech would be expected to stand farther away from the receivers of the

> Nonverbal immediacy behaviors on the part of physicians and other health care providers are very much related to patient satisfaction with care, and hence, outcomes.

message than a health care provider talking with a patient. There are certain distances that fall within a normal range of comfort for the parties communicating. Although there are cultural differences, most people are comfortable with certain distances in certain communication contexts. If, during a patient's visit to a physician, the physician entered the examining room, said hello, then sat down at the farthest point across the room from the patient, most patients would probably not find this distance comfortable. It would communicate indifference or discomfort on the part of the physician. On the other hand, if the physician entered the room, said hello, and then sat in a chair where his knees touched the patient's knees, this would not be comfortable either. It would be too intimate or immediate. The patient's own nonverbal cues (e.g., leaning back, crossing arms) would probably indicate this.

When a pharmacist is discussing health care matters with a patient, it is important that the physical distance between the two reflect the appropriate degree of immediacy. The distance should create some privacy (too far apart would mean your conversation would be audible to others) while at the same time not creating discomfort. Our patients will give us nonverbal cues when we stand too close. In North America, people in intimate or private conversations stand 6 to 18 inches apart.[6] This is what is generally comfortable. However, in some cultures, standing closer or farther away may be insulting. Physical distance can communicate the degree of caring or intimacy in a conversation.

Also, whether we sit or stand while talking to the patient communicates information about acceptance and caring. Sitting communicates that you are not going to rush things and places you in a position that is less intimidating to the patient. This is another reason why pharmacies are lowering their prescription counters to floor level. It promotes better communication.

The following example shows a pharmacist's use of proxemics: A patient who is obviously distressed tries to talk to the pharmacist, who is behind the counter. The counter presents a barrier to communication, so the pharmacist comes out from behind the counter and motions the patient to an area that is more private. This communicates caring, respect, and understanding to the patient.

Chronemics

In the United States we are extremely time conscious and are not used to waiting more than 5 minutes.[6] With a few exceptions (at nice restaurants, in physicians' offices), Americans resent waiting for long periods of time. Even a 15-minute wait, which is fairly common in many pharmacies, is viewed with impatience. It is important to convey value in the wait in order to reduce this negative view of waiting. This can be done by providing services worth waiting for (e.g., counseling, disease management), or it can be done by showing compassion and empathy. For example, consider the following scenario:

Patient: Fifteen minutes? Just to throw a few pills in a bottle? You've got to be kidding. I just had to wait almost an hour and a half at the doctor's office.

Pharmacist: That is a long time. I will get your medicine to you as quickly as I can. I do have two other patients ahead of you, and I want to be accurate with everyone's medicine. I do appreciate your patience.

Patient: I'm just sick of all this waiting. You people must think we have nothing better to do.

Pharmacist: I know that you have waited a long time today. I'm going to go ahead and get started so that it doesn't take any longer than necessary.

Notice in this situation that the pharmacist does not take the patient's frustration personally. Notice also that the pharmacist acknowledges the patient's complaint but does not take responsibility for the problem or attempt to solve it. The pharmacist is caring and compassionate but not willing to engage the patient in a debate.

Oculesics

Eye contact is very important in communicating understanding and caring. Direct eye contact communicates interest and attention. It helps us to gauge the truthfulness, intelligence, attitudes, and feelings of others. Our culture values direct eye contact (as long as it is not staring). In fact, we believe that people who won't look you directly in the eye are up to no good. There is a great deal of research showing that speakers who refuse to establish eye contact are perceived as ill at ease, insincere, or dishonest. Therefore, it is important to be aware of your own eye contact with patients when communicating with them.

Do you make a habit of doing other tasks when talking to patients? Do you find yourself looking more at a computer screen or medicine vials than at your patients? Not establishing eye contact while talking to a patient is likely to be distracting and communicates disinterest. Make it a point to establish good eye contact with your clients when talking to them. Also, keep in mind the patient's response to your eye contact. For example, by maintaining eye contact with the patient you are more likely to pick up nonverbal cues regarding whether the patient understands you. Many patients will say they understand when they truly don't, but patients' facial expressions, such as a raised eyebrow, often reveal confusion, misunderstanding, or uncertainty. These important cues can be missed by pharmacists who do not take the time to maintain eye contact. Although it is generally true that direct eye contact may have negative consequences in negative or threatening situations, and lack of eye contact often communicates indifference or inattention, the amount of eye contact should depend on the patient's response. If the patient reacts uncomfortably to your direct eye contact, looking away occasionally may be a good idea.

Haptics

Touch can be extremely important in communicating caring to a patient. Touch has generally been found to reduce tension, affect rapport, and enhance the therapeutic abilities of the health professional.[7] The use of touch is very much dependent on the emotional context, the relationship between the patient and the pharmacist, and how comfortable the pharmacist and patient are about the use of touch. Anglo-Americans tend to use touch less often than Italian-Americans and Afro-Americans.[6] Therefore, touch may be interpreted very differently among these groups. Although different groups tend to use more touch, there are few cultural standards for touch. Therefore, touch needs to be used with caution.

According to some studies, touch by a health care professional can be interpreted as superficial or demeaning if it is used too often during a conversation or an encounter. This could be true when touch is used as a substitute for verbally expressing true caring and understanding or when touch is used to diminish the importance of a problem without appropriate expression in words. For example, if a patient is discussing the amount of pain he is experiencing from his arthritis and the physician pats him on the back, this type of touch may be interpreted as placating but not caring. The same touch with the words "Let's see if we can't get you some medicine that will help with this pain" would be interpreted quite differently. In addition, when touch is used with a new patient, it is often misinterpreted or viewed with caution.

Moreover, touch should not be used if the patient or health care provider is uncomfortable with it. The health care provider should be especially sensitive to the verbal and nonverbal cues of the patient. Posture that pulls away or a startled look is a good indication that this is not comfortable for the patient. If you are not comfortable being touched or touching others, it is best to not force a touch. Sincere words will do just as well. Touching is viewed as a rather intimate gesture in our culture and, as such, should be used carefully and cautiously.

Kinesics

Kinesics concerns itself with body movement in communication. This includes movement of the head, arms, legs, eyes, and so on. Body movement can have a profound impact on the way a message is communicated and interpreted. If I look at you and say "way to go" but my head is shaking "no," no is the message you will likely believe. The message will be interpreted as sarcasm. It is vitally important that both nonverbal body movements and tone of voice (vocalics—more on this later) match the verbal message. Congruence is essential. Haase and Tepper[8] found that, especially in counseling situations, highly empathic messages are undermined by inconsistent or incongruent nonverbal messages, including body movements (looking away, being distracted), voice tone (flat affect, indifference), and body position (standing, back to person).

It should be noted that kinesics is very much tied to cultural norms. The gesture of pointing to someone to indicate that his or her prescription is ready is perfectly normal in our culture. That same gesture is indicated only for calling dogs in some African countries. Extending a hand to introduce yourself to a patient is perfectly normal in our culture. Done with the wrong hand, it may be considered an insult in some Middle Eastern cultures (the "wrong" hand is used only for wiping oneself after defecating). So, although some gestures are the same across many cultures, different cultures can give very different meanings to the same gestures.

Being aware of your own gestures and body movements is very important. It can help you to congruently communicate the intended meaning of your verbal statements.

Objectics

This refers to both the use and choice of objects in communication. One very important object is the clothing we choose to wear. It can communicate a great deal about us. Are the clothes in style? Are they ironed or wrinkled? Do the colors go together? How does the pharmacist distinguish himself or herself from the rest of the staff in the pharmacy? Does the pharmacist wear a professional coat that is a different color and has an identifying name badge or symbol indicating that he or she is a pharmacist? It is important for patients to understand to whom they are talking so that they don't waste time and effort and feel embarrassed if they tell ancillary personnel information that was intended only for a health professional. Clothes certainly can communicate expertise to the patient by way of specific identifiers.

In addition to clothing, other objects communicate different messages. Is there an area in the pharmacy where patients can sit and wait? If so, this communicates sensitivity to the clients. Are the chairs comfortable? Is the waiting area clean? Are there reading materials in the waiting area? Are they health related, or is there a variety of both health-related and non-health-related materials? Are there popular magazines to read? Are they out-of-date? All of these things communicate different things to patients. Are the objects surrounding your pharmacy communicating the message you want to communicate? Many pharmacies sell items that are not health related. These may include cigarettes, cosmetics, greeting cards, household items (e.g., paper towels, toilet paper, glass cleaners), and candy. Does selling these items confuse the patient about what our primary intent is as a health care provider? Is selling these items consistent with the health image you are trying to convey? Quite frankly, why would any health care provider sell items such as cigarettes and tobacco, which are clearly deleterious to health? Profit simply does not justify the sale of these items in a pharmacy. This is a primary example of how important objectics can be in communicating an image. In moving toward pharmaceutical care, pharmacies may need to reconsider the items they sell and the effects of those items on the image conveyed.

Vocalics

This involves the use of the human voice in communication. It involves both tone and pitch. Think about this sentence: "I really like it when you come in on time for your medicine." That same sentence can be said very differently, depending on pitch, tone, and emphasis. Said blandly, the statement may not have much impact. Said with enthusiasm and emphasis on certain words, the meaning changes: "I *really like it* when you come in on time for you medicine!" This is encouraging. However, if this same sentence is said sarcastically to a patient who is 7 days late in getting his medicine, the meaning changes again: "I *really* like it when you come in on time." This, said with a look of disapproval, would be belittling to the patient.

The human voice communicates much to the receiver. This is especially true when communication takes place over the telephone. Research indicates that personality is inferred through the sound of the voice. Often the interpretation is inaccurate because of preconceived ideas we have about different types of voices. We may think of someone with a deep voice as being wise or large, for example. What this should tell us is that we need to be sure that the meaning we intend is communicated clearly, especially when talking on the telephone.

> We often focus on the words spoken, but 93% of the meaning of a message is derived from nonverbal cues. It is very important that there is congruence between verbal and nonverbal cues.

Pulling It Together

Scenario: Mrs. Monroe is obviously distressed. She has just learned that she has skin cancer.

Proxemics: The pharmacist steps from behind the counter and motions Mrs. Monroe to a more private area. Mrs. Monroe indicates that the physician was confusing when she talked about the possible side effects of the medication.

Oculesics: The pharmacist goes over the possible side effects and explains what Mrs. Monroe should do if they occur. The pharmacist observes that Mrs. Monroe looks confused. So, he stops and asks her if she understands. She says she does. Even though she replies that she understands, he provides a more thorough, detailed explanation. After this explanation, Mrs. Monroe's facial expressions indicate that she understands.

Kinesics: The pharmacist makes sure that his body movements and facial expressions are congruent with his words. That is, when he says he is concerned, he looks concerned.

Vocalics: During the conversation, the pharmacist varies his tone, rate, and volume. For example, the pharmacist noticed that Mrs. Monroe tended to whisper the word *cancer*. Therefore, he also lowered his voice whenever he used the word. The pharmacist used a soft, calm, and even tone throughout the conversation as a means of comfort.

Haptics: At one point during the conversation, the pharmacist placed his hand on Mrs. Monroe's hand, looked into her eyes, and said in a sincere tone, "I want to help you through this."

Summary of Nonverbal Immediacy

Nonverbal communication is an important factor in conveying the meaning in a message. Verbal and nonverbal messages need to be congruent, since the nonverbal message is the one that is generally believed. It is not enough to accurately perceive a patient's feelings and to communicate that understanding verbally. Physical distance, posture, objects in the environment, voice tone, and gestures can all change the meaning of the message. The most effective counselors are the ones whose nonverbal messages are congruent with their verbal messages.

Questions for Reflection

1. Congruence between verbal and nonverbal messages is essential. What can you do to achieve message congruence?
2. In what ways can you create more immediate messages for patients? How might you improve what you are currently doing?
3. When is it appropriate to touch a patient? When is it inappropriate? Should you touch a patient even if you are uncomfortable about doing so?
4. What role does culture play in nonverbal communication?
5. What should you do if a patient does not want to be more immediate in his or her communication with you?

References

1. Wiener M, Mehrabian A. *Language within Language: Immediacy, a Channel in Verbal Communication.* New York: Appleton-Century-Crofts; 1968.
2. Cupach WR., Metts S. *Facework.* Thousand Oaks, Calif: Sage Publications; 1994.
3. Von Friederichs-Fitzwater MM. *The Analysis of Verbal Immediacy in the Communication of Care Providers and Terminally Ill Patients.* Ann Arbor, Mich: UMI Dissertation Information Service; 1989.
4. Conlee C, Olvera J. The relationships among physician nonverbal immediacy and measures of patient satisfaction with physician care. *Commun Rep.* 1993;6(1):25–34.
5. Mehrabian A. *Silent Messages.* Belmont, Calif: Wadsworth Publishing; 1971.
6. McCroskey JC. *An Introduction to Rhetorical Communication.* Englewood Cliffs, NJ: Prentice Hall; 1982.
7. DiMatteo MR, DiNicola DD. *Achieving Patient Compliance.* New York: Pergamon Press; 1982.
8. Haase RF, Tepper DT. Nonverbal components of empathic communication. *J Counsel Psychol.* 1972;19:417–24.

Index